PRAISE FOR

The Mindful Addict

"When I picked up Tom's book and started reading it,
I couldn't put it down. This is an outstanding book and promises
to enrich anyone's recovery regardless of whether they are a newcomer
or a long-timer. Tom's inspiring journey, his gut-wrenching honesty,
and his commitment to living a conscious and mindful life reveal
the true nature of the process of recovery.

The seeds to Tom's recovery were planted well before he put
together any serious time clean. It has been stated that recovery is
dependent upon a spiritual experience set on a pedestal of hopelessness.
Clearly Tom's pain and suffering spawned a spiritual awakening. But
he didn't do it alone. In recovery we learn that 'We can do what I can't.'
Tom had a very special person in his life, Flobird. Through Tom's
story you will meet this remarkable woman. I like to think of her
as Tom's spiritual midwife. She and many others helped Tom build
a very strong foundation for his recovery.

Tom has taken his spiritual wounds and his addiction, and
transformed them into sacred wounds. This is the direct result
of his commitment to go to any lengths to stay clean and his
willingness and courage to listen to the voice within.

Tom has given us a wonderful gift in *The Mindful Addict* by sharing
his experience, fears, strength, and hope. Thank you, Tom!"

–Allen Berger, Ph.D.
Author of *12 Stupid Things That Mess Up Recovery: Avoiding
Relapse through Self-Awareness and Right Action* and *12 Smart Things
to Do When the Booze and Drugs Are Gone: Choosing Emotional
Sobriety through Self-Awareness and Right Action*

• • •

"I picked up Tom Catton's manuscript one afternoon and decided to read the book right away. I found it engrossing and insightful. I finished the book that evening, and I can vouch for its authenticity as I was one of Flobird's 'traveling birds.' Tom offers hope and inspiration about how to navigate through life before and after recovery. May many lives be touched by Tom's journey and learn the meaning of being happy and grateful in recovery and in service to others."

–Reverend Deborah Knowles
Unity Church of Kona-Kohala, Kona, Hawaii

• • •

"Everyone's life is a drama; Tom Catton's is a true adventure. Not only is *The Mindful Addict* an adventure in recovery; it is an adventure in discovery. What Tom finds, and what he helps all of us find, is the glorious truth about ourselves and the world in which we live. Tom knows what it is to hit rock bottom, and he has graced us all with a book that is completely rock solid."

–Rabbi Rami Shapiro
Author of *Recovery—The Sacred Art:*
The Twelve Steps as Spiritual Practice

• • •

"So much is made of the question 'Are we always in a state of recovery, or can we ever fully recover from addiction?' With *The Mindful Addict*, Tom Catton does as good a job as I have seen of dispatching this meaningless question. Here is a book that will give you the practical tools you need to live fully in the moment, a moment that is eternally revealing itself to us. All we need do is pay attention. Simple, but far from easy, of course. But if you are serious about recovery, this is a path worth choosing. And I highly recommend Tom Catton as one of your guides."

–Thom Rutledge
Author of *Embracing Fear: How to Turn*
What Scares Us into Our Greatest Gift

"Many search for spiritual enlightenment, but few have survived the path Tom Catton details in *The Mindful Addict*. This is a beautiful tale of one soul's long journey back from the brink of a life immersed in alcohol and drugs. Along the way, Tom discovers the key to his survival is complete surrender to a higher source. I highly recommend surrendering to *The Mindful Addict* and letting the awakening of your spirit begin as well."

–Randolph J. Rogers
Author of *The Key of Life:*
A Metaphysical Investigation

THE
MINDFUL
ADDICT

A Memoir of
the Awakening
of a Spirit

BY TOM CATTON

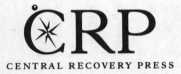

CENTRAL RECOVERY PRESS

CENTRAL RECOVERY PRESS

Central Recovery Press (CRP) is committed to publishing exceptional materials addressing addiction treatment, recovery, and behavioral health care, including original and quality books, audio/visual communications, and Web-based new media. Through a diverse selection of titles, it seeks to impact the behavioral health care field with a broad range of unique resources for professionals, recovering individuals, and their families.

For more information, visit www.centralrecoverypress.com.

Central Recovery Press, Las Vegas, NV 89129
© 2010 by Tom Catton

ISBN-13: 978-0-9818482-7-3
ISBN-10: 0-9818482-7-3

16 15 14 13 12 11 10   1 2 3 4 5

Publisher: Central Recovery Press
              3371 N. Buffalo Drive
              Las Vegas, NV 89129

Cover design and interior by Sara Streifel, Think Creative Design

Editor's Note: *The Mindful Addict* is based on real events to the best of the author's recollection. To protect the anonymity of those mentioned in this book, some names and identifying details have been changed.

To my loving wife Bea Austin. To my daughter Celeste and son-in-law Joe, and to my son Josh and his lovely wife Khym. To my six wonderful grandchildren, Sage, Hayley, Sydney, Kyan, Hunter, and Shea. To my parents. And, of course, to Flobird.

TABLE OF

CONTENTS

FOREWORD

The Mindful Addict isn't the typical recovery memoir. Where most such stories start to fizzle out after the hero emerges from the drama and horror of addiction, Tom's just gets going. Sure, his years of drug addiction are compelling to read about, but it's in his recovery that the story takes off. When he got clean as the sixties turned to the seventies, drugs and charismatic hucksters pervaded the spiritual scene, and his guide into recovery, Flobird, reads more like one of those trippy cult leaders than any twelve-step sponsor I've ever heard of—but she *is* in recovery, and that makes all the difference.

Tom is a kind of spiritual everyman, seeking out Mother Teresa and Ram Dass, taking on celibacy and poverty, hanging out at Edgar Cayce's library and Yogananda's ashram. Like a character in some eighteenth-century picaresque novel, Tom takes us from one illuminating moment to another, guided only by his longing to serve, to grow, and to experience spiritual bliss and connection. Along the way, his outward innocence hides an inner wisdom. Never claiming to be a guru, Tom nonetheless teaches us through his experiences and through the broad-ranging insights that develop over a lifetime of recovery and spiritual practice. And just when you think his story is ready to fizzle, aging and illness bring more lessons.

His determination is remarkable, a testament to the twelve-step principle of "showing up" that he embodies. When I first met Tom, he told me he wanted to write the story of his life. When he sent me his early attempts, I was skeptical. Here was a guy with a high school education who was recovering from brain surgery—how much could you expect from him? But with true humility, he set out to learn what it would take to create a great book. He showed tenacity and a willingness to be a beginner that most people—especially those with decades of clean time—could never muster. And even though I followed the process and knew how committed he was, I was still amazed by the quality of the end result. *The Mindful Addict* is a book that is going to touch a lot of people, ultimately not because of the glamour of Tom's life, but because of the authenticity of his love and the power of his message. As Tom says, he's "out living and loving life to the fullest in the present moment," and after reading this book, that's what you're going to want to do too.

–**Kevin Griffin**

Author of *One Breath at a Time: Buddhism and the Twelve Steps* and *A Burning Desire: Dharma God & the Path of Recovery*

PREFACE

My name is Tom, and I'm an addict of the hopeless variety. This is my story and my adventure. I was catapulted into another dimension, transported from a life full of fear and separateness to a life full of miracles and synchronicity, a life that is now overflowing with love and intimacy.

Since October 20, 1971, I have followed the spiritual path of twelve-step programs. The teachings I have learned throughout my life's journey of personal challenges began in a state of hopeless addiction. But my teachers, studies, and experiences on a variety of spiritual paths have led me to believe in the possibility—and simplicity—of finding true happiness. Living life to the fullest, with an attitude of gratitude, has become my mantra over the years. It has led me to experience life with a true joy for living, despite external circumstances.

This book shows how, through meditation, a person who had no prior training came to have his life profoundly changed by the practice. Meditation teaches us to always follow our inner guidance and stay present in the moment. Along with offering love and service to others, meditation leads to a fulfilling life. We can be happy right here, right now—not if and when our specific desires materialize.

What I share here is my experience. I do not claim to be any kind of expert or teacher within the twelve-step arena, and although I find myself attracted to Buddhism, there will be no formal teachings in this book. There are numerous books on Buddhism and twelve-step programs. My simple goal is to share what has worked and is currently working in my life. I'm drawn to the school of Theravada Buddhism, from where the now-popular Vipassana practice of meditation stems.

The word "mindfulness" will be mentioned throughout the book. Mindfulness comes from the Sanskrit word *sati*, which means basic awareness, and the word *smirti*, meaning "to come back" to awareness when the mind starts to stray. Simply, it all means "Pay attention to what is." We need not acquire a black belt in meditation, visit seven higher realms, or have direct contact with the angels around us. We just have to be present and constantly give of ourselves as we walk through our lives. That's how we truly discover that our serenity is only and always a breath away.

I invite you to join me on this journey. The spiritual path is open to each of us. Although it contains many bumps and some darkness, we will walk it together, and we will always find our way to the light.

ACKNOWLEDGMENTS

There have been countless people and experiences that ultimately led to the writing of this book. They are too numerous to mention by name, but I am thankful for them all. As I write this, I am reminded that I am no mere spectator of coincidence, but a participant in fate.

First I must thank my co-conspirator on this path: my loving wife, Bea Austin, who always stayed focused on the process and reminded me that I was led to write, and that is all I needed to do—write! The guidance was always about the writing and not the result. The people who directly helped with this book are listed and incriminated below. This is my story, and I'm sticking to it.

This is how it all played out:

While at a meditation workshop weekend in 2007, I mentioned to my friend Lucy Jokiel that I was writing a book. At that moment as we ascended the stairs, she said, "Tom, I will help you by doing some editing." That brief exchange was the beginning that led to the first draft. Then George Krzyminski came along and put his helpful touch on some of the earlier drafts. My daughter, Celeste Barcia, took precious time from her busy life to help me go over those first tentative writings.

My dharma teacher, Kevin Griffin, offered constructive comments, and then was kind enough to introduce me to Lisa Fugard. Lisa went through the manuscript and marked it up, revealing even more territories on the map. Following her skilled guidance and encouraging direction gave me the bravery to "clean house" and start a complete rewrite.

I feel compelled to send much thankfulness and credit to Christy Maxwell and Dan Brown, who both stayed with me through the final draft of this book. Together they added much of their hearts and helped bring the book to its victory lap.

I'd like to thank my publisher, Central Recovery Press. Without their commitment and belief in this book, it would still be inside my computer, and just a dream. Thanks for making it a reality.

And finally, a very special thanks to all my friends on Facebook. As I finished the writing, I would find myself periodically posting excerpts from the book. Your loving responses and encouragement kept me at the keyboard in those long last hours. Namaste.

INTRODUCTION

3:45 a.m., February 10, 1968, Kaneohe, Hawaii. A tall, thin woman looking much older than her fifty-two years sits up in bed, meditating. A cup of coffee rests on her nightstand, and a cigarette glows in the dark. She listens in silence to the small voice within, her shadow standing guard as she sits in the stillness, becoming one with the calm. Flobird meditates for several hours every morning, a habit she picked up in 1960 while getting into twelve-step recovery.

She lives each day by the spiritual guidance she receives during meditation and diligently records the messages in her journal. Writing becomes automatic, a prayer in ink, and the spirit guiding her pen to identify her next assignment. At times her dialogue with God is intense, and at times she questions the assignment; but she always steps into the unknown and does exactly as her spirit guides her.

On this particular morning, Flobird's meditation leads her to the North Shore of Oahu, about forty miles from Kaneohe. She hops into "Redbird," her Fiat, and drives to the Sunset Beach area. There she finds a four-bedroom, completely furnished, wood-framed home nestled under the trees right on the oceanfront. Guided by an inner direction, she reaches above the doorjamb, locates the key, unlocks the door, and enters. Coincidentally, I live next door.

During the winter months, the waves on the North Shore are huge. This is the only time they break with massive force, and they must be at least twenty feet high before they are considered surfable by the locals. The energy from just one such large wave as it comes crashing down is breathtaking, and the salt spray can be seen in the air for miles.

At night, the roaring waves sound like thunder or a gigantic gong echoing across the oceans from some unknown temple. Often they become so enormous that they wash over the highway. Sometimes these monster waves can even level houses in their path.

The North Shore community is relatively small, and everyone knows one another. Today, Haleiwa, the main village, is a bustling town sought out by tourists from all over the world who come to watch or surf the killer waves; but back in the 1960s, it had only two grocery stores and a bank.

This time and place was magical for those of us fortunate enough to live there. The community was dominated by surfers from around the world who competed at the world's most famous surf spots, which dotted the five-mile stretch of coastline. There were also so-called hippies searching for enlightenment through the use of drugs, including LSD and hashish, which were believed to lead to spiritual illumination. Some of these drug-using hippies were in both categories: They surfed and took a lot of drugs, but they were ultimately looking for something greater. *That was me.*

In the early morning hours of this day, I was startled awake by the sound of a car on our lane. With a clarity entirely unfamiliar to me in the breaking dawn, I gazed out the window and saw a tiny red Fiat pull up to the vacant house next door. I watched curiously as a strange woman got out and walked calmly up to the house as if she indisputably belonged, as if placed there by mystical entitlement. I had no idea this event would change my life forever.

CHAPTER ONE

THE
BEGINNING

As I held the match under the spoon, heating up the water to help the white powder dissolve, the anticipation of shooting pure methedrine into my veins caused a feeling of electricity to race through my sleepless and deprived body. I had been awake for three days, and every time I fixed, I told myself I would never do it again. My wife was asleep. It was 2 a.m., and the world was quiet. But this quietness did not exist inside my head. Anxiety, fear, and separation plagued me like demons. I had moved beyond any human level of desperation. I would have settled for hell.

Sitting in the bathroom with a soft light on, I tied a belt around my arm and pumped up my veins. Gently, almost sexually, I tapped the top of the syringe until I saw blood back up—the sign the needle is in the vein. I had become so intimate with my loneliness through the process of fixing dope. How did I get here? I squeezed the syringe, and the rush overtook me as my hair stood on end. My using had become a madman's paradox: The more I used to get further out of myself, the deeper I found myself locked within. I created a new prison with every hit.

At the time we lived on the Venice Canals in Venice, California. It was the summer of 1967, the time of love-ins, Tim Leary, LSD, and free love. We were hippies, extending a childhood dream of blissful states, resonating love, and dancing in the streets. So why was I in this bathroom alone? Where was the love? I was not free. My flowers had turned brown. The garden was in decay. What had happened since the first time I picked up a drink and then continued on to drugs? Drugs and alcohol had initially given me relief from the separateness I felt. Even though I had come from a loving middle-class family, I never felt I fit in. Drugs helped ease my feelings of disconnection, so I continued to use them, seeking relief from those feelings that had haunted me my entire life. The dope brought a softness I had mistaken as peace. The drugs had simply silenced me.

As I removed the needle from my arm and felt the drug rush through my body, touching every cell within, I sat there with the syringe in my hand, blood dripping on the floor, waiting for relief that did not seem to come. How many times had I repeated this scene? Again I found myself high and trembling on uneasy knees. Again I found myself praying and in pain. I had always believed in a God, so I prayed to be released, not even sure from what or to where. My hands shook as I folded them to pray, the way I had been taught. Yet now, kneeling on the cold tile of the bathroom floor, my devotion seemed destroyed. Fear and despair were all I knew.

I sat there and reflected back almost twenty years earlier, on the memory of my first day of school, when the feelings of isolation and separation began. I was four-and-a-half years old. We lived in a small rented house on about an acre of land in Mar Vista, California, which was only a few miles from the house in Venice. Mom packed my lunchbox and loaded my sister in the baby carriage, and we walked about ten minutes up our alley to the school.

Our dog, Dane, followed closely behind. I looked around at the familiar surroundings, but everything appeared strange. It seemed like my life was changing, and I didn't know how to express what I was feeling. I wanted to say, "No, Mom, I can't do this. I can't leave you, Cindy, and Dane. Mom, I'm too little to do this." But my mouth didn't form these words. On the short walk, I seemingly slipped through a portal into a world that may have looked the same, but where I did not belong.

As we walked into the schoolyard, kids were running around having fun, and they all seemed to know each other. I knew immediately I was different and hid behind Mom's floral skirt as we walked into the classroom. I looked down and studied the checkered tile floor. Desks were lined up in perfect order, and a blackboard took up most of one wall. All kinds of paper decorations and colored objects hung on the other walls. As kids rushed in and happily sat at their desks, I felt overwhelmed by feelings of sheer terror I had never experienced. All I could do was beg my mom not to leave.

Of course, she had to go, and I was left alone in this perplexing new world with peculiar people. As the teacher wrote on the blackboard, the other students nodded their heads in understanding, writing down our daily activities. But I was frozen, paralyzed within, to the extent of hearing the sound coming out of the teacher's mouth—but the words were in a language I could not understand. The disease of addiction—which is rooted in separation—had started in little Tommy's life. This was the moment in which I clearly remember encountering my first feelings of separation and not fitting in, feelings I later discovered are nearly universal for addicts. Little did I know these unpleasant feelings would intensify and cause me and others great pain as I grew older.

Along with the LSD movement happening in the sixties, eastern philosophy had become popular in the U.S. While living in Southern California I would go to the Self-Realization Fellowship (SRF), an organization that taught meditation. It had a meditation chapel and bookstore where you could purchase all sorts of books about the spiritual life. SRF was about a mile up Sunset Boulevard from Coast Highway 1. The sprawling grounds were home to a lake, with beautiful gardens dotting the hillsides that sloped down to the path surrounding it. People visited to walk the garden paths and to find a sanctuary in the middle of the busy city. It became my place for a psychedelic experience, taking LSD as I strolled amongst the devotees.

SRF was founded by Paramahansa Yogananda, the author of *Autobiography of a Yogi.* I read this book in 1966. That was my first experience with eastern philosophy, and I was strongly drawn to the book and its spiritual teachings. Yogananda describes growing up in India, traveling in the Himalaya mountains, and the many gurus he encountered on his journeys.

This philosophy seemed to dovetail with the LSD movement, including the belief that the love and light that exist within everyone lead to being one with God. It didn't include a concept of hell or the devil. Instead, it focused on the importance of karma—the idea that whatever you put out, you will get back. My heart was immediately attracted to these beliefs. My soul was craving to find its way home.

SRF offered meditation lessons through the mail, so I readily subscribed. After shooting methedrine or taking any variety of assorted drugs, I would try to meditate, but with 70,000 drug-induced thoughts a minute rushing through my head, I was unable to find the way to the one breath the lessons described. From the time I started using drugs, I experimented with many different chemicals. LSD, pot, hashish, and mescaline were all used by our generation for spiritual reasons; at least that is what I told myself.

4

Despite my best intentions, I inevitably returned to the destructive cycle of shooting drugs and taking mind-altering pills. Today it's clear to me that although I was constantly searching for a spiritual solution, drugs failed to lessen my emotional pain. But as an addict, I was unable to stop using drugs and rely solely on meditation and the teachings of popular gurus. Drugs had become part of my solution, and it was impossible to see that these mind-numbing, painkilling agents were actually hindering my ability to connect with the spirit. I was unable to hear the words "You have a drug problem." This was the 1960s. The only "problem" was that not everyone used drugs. My using had brought on the rationalization that was pulling me to the bottom spiritually, physically, and emotionally.

The Venice Canals were made up of waterways that ran parallel to each other, like the actual Venice canals in Italy. In the 1920s this was considered a high-end place to live, but by the 1960s it was more or less run down. Lots of so-called hippies were living in the houses lining each canal. Today this area has been renovated to its previous high-dollar real estate status. The entrance of our small, stucco house faced a waterway. The only way to approach the front of the house was via a small boat. An alley ran behind the house so that it could be approached by car. I was constantly strung out and sleeping very little because I was shooting so much speed. Nevertheless, I continued to study my SRF lessons. A line in one of the lessons read: *When the student is ready, the teacher will appear.* When I read this, it was as if a neon sign flashed those words in my mind, and in the months to come I never forgot that statement.

Using speed and not sleeping, I felt more and more hopeless. I peered, bleary-eyed, out the windows all night, watching shadow people moving through the streets and bouncing off the sides of houses. Were they warning me? Protecting me? Or after me? I believed my house was being watched and my phone was tapped. Sometimes I rowed my small boat up and down the canals all night, the water reflecting the moonlight as I glided across the glassy surface, with only the sound of the oars as they splashed in the water. It was a romantic scene. The key problem was that my wife was asleep, leaving only me and my German shepherd dogs in the rowboat to guard against nefarious forces unknown. As I floated by, the darkened shoreline houses appeared almost peaceful, a feeling I had long ago lost. When I drifted by a house with muted light shining through a window, I wondered, "Are they like me? What is running through their veins?" The drugs and sleep deprivation made me feel completely paranoid, although some of my paranoia was probably well-founded.

One day some friends were over, and we were using drugs. While looking out the window, I saw a nondescript black sedan that looked like a narc's car slowing down near our house. My intuition turned to alarm, and I yelled for everyone to clear out. Everyone dove out the front windows and ran down the canals. I ran out into the alley with my two dogs and watched, calmly, as the narcs got out of their car and began walking up to my house. Without forethought, I suddenly jumped directly in their faces, which curtailed their surprise attack. They just stood there, stunned, before returning to their car and driving away.

Shaken by the incident, I knew things were getting out of hand on the canals. Even with my shattered emotions, I was able to hear an inner voice. It told me I could no longer keep running in place. I had to move. I went to my friend Wes's house and told him I thought we should leave town. Wes was strung out also, so we packed up a bunch of drugs (not speed, because I had vowed to stop using it) and determined the best plan to get out of town quickly. I turned to my parents, who knew what was going on in my life. I had encouraged their denial of my condition, but my behavior and the circumstances of my life soon broke through the façade that I was okay. They had found drugs in my dresser drawers when I was living at home, and a syringe had dropped out of my dirty clothes once when I went to use their washer. So in their own desperation to help me, and not knowing what else to do, my parents gave Wes and me money to fly back to Hawaii. I had been going back and forth between Hawaii and California since my first visit in 1962 when I was kicked out of the twelfth grade.

I started surfing in 1959. Living in Southern California, it seemed like the thing to do. Attending Santa Monica High, I was only about four blocks from the beach, so my surfboard resided in the back of my 1955 Ford station wagon at all times. Surfing at lunchtime or before school became a daily routine.

My next-door neighbor Ron and I would head up to Malibu Point before school. I remember perfect five- to six-foot glassy waves and the water shining like a mirror as we paddled out at dawn. On beautiful, sunny days, with perfect waves and a gentle offshore breeze, I was in total bliss. Taking off on a wave on my nine-foot-three-inch Velzy and Jacobs board and turning in to a wall of water made everything else disappear. While surfing, I was completely in the present moment. All my problems, stress, and anything weighing on my mind were completely dismissed. It was just me, the water, and the sound of the surfboard slipping across the wave's face, like a rock skipping across the surface of a windless lake.

I would look up as Ronnie was paddling out on his knees. As our eyes met, no words were necessary. He knew what was going on inside me, and we just smiled at this beautiful moment—the perfect wave and the flawless ride. During these moments in the ocean, I understood connectivity to myself, to others, and to nature. Although the ride usually lasted for only seconds, it seemed like an eternity.

Experiences like this bring a person completely into the moment. Later I learned from my meditation practice that being in the moment is where real happiness is found. Today, as I move through my life, I practice being in the present in all of my activities—it's like riding that wave.

By the time I entered high school, the separateness had become a regular part of my life. I was extremely shy and unsure of myself in unfamiliar situations, especially with girls, and there was no way I could ever ask anyone out on a date. My self-doubt was enormous, but once I discovered getting loaded, a whole new world opened up to me.

My parents were social drinkers who had booze in our house for get-togethers when their friends came over for the evening. I remember my first drinking experience. My friends and I filled quart jars with a little vodka and some bourbon and scotch—a nice toxic mixture. Then we drank it. As the alcohol went down my throat, it burned and gagged me. I could barely get the stuff down. But at the same time, this wonderful feeling of warmth surged throughout my body. For the first time, I felt truly okay. I felt complete.

I got exceedingly drunk, threw up everywhere, and woke up the next day with a terrible hangover. I didn't remember much about the night before, but I sure wanted to do it again—and really soon. Alcohol had magically taken away that terrifying feeling of separation that had become a powerful part of my life. The aftermath the following day left me shaky, dehydrated, and torn down, but it seemed like a fair trade for that momentary state of self-assured bliss. What another may have viewed as degradation, I simply saw as part of the experience— jagged around the edges, but smooth enough for me to endure.

So the adventure had started, and there was no turning back. I thought it was a marvelous experience. From a shy person who was too timid to ask a woman for a date, I had turned into a wild man who went to parties and ended up running around naked and out of my mind. I began to feel connected to a world from which I had previously felt so separated. Alcohol had become my friend, and my world was okay when I was hanging out with this new friend. I began to develop a sort of selective amnesia, my mind forgetting all the nightmarish scenes that would ensue. I was learning the art of bargaining with myself. Or was it the gift of denial?

I was open to anything that got me high. My new principle to live by was: Try anything once, and if the resulting damage is in any way negotiable, a second time will settle any doubts. I soon began sniffing glue. I became a regular at hobby shops, buying model airplane glue and squirting the glue into a sock.

Surfing and getting drunk or loaded went together for me at that time. The drugs and alcohol did for me what I couldn't do for myself. I used my station wagon for surfing and dating, with the backseat in a down position at all times. This served two functions: It was great for surfing trips when people had to ride in the back with the boards, and it was great for date night at the drive-in movies. Now I had the courage to ask girls out, but I had absolutely no social or dating skills. Where other guys may have used tried-and-true standbys like flowers or a serenade from a guitar to court a girl, I would bring out the beer and glue socks. It's easy to imagine what a healthy teenage boy wants to do while on a date with a beautiful girl at the drive-in. My problem was that when I got close to making out with my date, I would stick a glue rag between our mouths and say, "Try this." I always wondered why the girl didn't want to go out with me again. The disconnect between reality and how I was starting to operate only deepened, and the line between myself and "them" was unmistakable.

So drugs became my best friend, especially grass and pills. Chemicals were now my confidant, seductress, lifestyle, and destination all in one. I remember the first time I took a stimulant, those little white cross pills called Benzedrine, or "bennies." My then-girlfriend Cindi, a beautiful Asian girl, lived about twenty miles north in Malibu, so I took three bennies and started driving up the Coast Highway. All of a sudden they kicked in, and my first thought (being a true addict) was: "I have to have a thousand of these things." The second thought was: "Where is a hitchhiker when you need one?" I was so wired out by the pills that I was talking to myself nonstop.

I would have been a graduate of the class of 1962 at Santa Monica High School, but by the eleventh grade I was slipping away from student life. Consistent with my surfer lifestyle, I began growing my hair long, resulting in frequent expulsions from school. I also missed many classes to go surfing at lunchtime, often not returning to school, or sometimes I went surfing before school and didn't go to class at all that day. Teachers, classrooms, and a formal education seemed like trivial things I had moved beyond. I had evolved into a creature who spent his days surfing the sunlit waves and his nights stoned under the moon- and starlit sky.

The summer before my senior year, school officials told my parents I had to get a haircut before I would be allowed to attend classes. I thought, "That's great, let me just quit now." But my parents wouldn't go for that, so I got a haircut and was allowed to enter the twelfth grade. I had already given up on school and reacted to everything with total rebellion: missing or getting expelled from classes, talking back to my teachers, not doing homework. I worked diligently at dropping out. My plan worked. Eventually, I just reported to the dean's office in place of certain classes, and finally I was kicked out of school for good.

What does a typical California surfer do after being kicked out of school? He heads for a surfing heaven like Hawaii, which is exactly what I did in April of 1962. It was my first trip to the islands, and I stayed on Oahu for about a month. I arrived late at night and was picked up by some friends I had surfed with in California who had arrived in Hawaii a few weeks before me. As I stepped off the plane, the warm, balmy breeze swept over me, and the fragrant air was especially sweet; this tropical environment felt so good. This place felt like home. The spell of the islands had been cast.

Early the next morning, I headed for the ocean, strolling through the empty streets of Waikiki. Watching the coconut trees swaying in the morning breeze, I walked across the sand and dipped my foot into the water. It was like a heated pool. I dove in, and my body immediately tingled with the warmth of the water washing over me. In contrast to the shockingly cold California ocean, this water seemed to embrace me. The ocean's heavier salt content kept my body buoyant and stung my eyes as the water rolled down my face. I had played in the ocean my whole life, but this first experience in the waters of

Hawaii was like stepping through a portal into another consciousness. It was as if part of my being had been hypnotized, and the magic waters shook me awake. I knew in that moment I wanted to spend the rest of my life in the islands.

That first trip I stayed in Hawaii for a month, just surfing and lying on the beach. I spent the summer months back in California at Malibu Beach doing more of the same—surfing and getting high. I returned to Hawaii for a second trip in December of 1962 for another month of surfing.

Despite my love for the ocean, during that period of time in Santa Monica, including the two trips to Hawaii, I became hopelessly lost. The drugs had already quit working, but I continued to use them. The feelings of self-doubt, fear, and separation had returned. Getting high was no longer effective in deadening my emotional pain.

In the summer of 1963, I went back to Hawaii for my third trip. I landed with a surfboard and about fifteen dollars in my pocket. I didn't work for the entire four months I was there. Being only nineteen at the time, having quit school and learned no vocational skills, and not knowing how to even look for a job, I knew nothing but this lifestyle of surfing and using drugs. I would break into a car on the street late at night, curl up on the backseat and fall asleep, and then wake up the next morning and head for the nearest gas station to use the restroom. The rest of the day, I surfed and begged for money on the street. I was homeless long before it became as commonplace as it is today.

We certainly look different on the outside than we feel on the inside. There was something adventurous about being a surf bum, spending days in the sun and ocean and nights at parties. Tom Catton, I'm sure, was acquiring a certain reputation as I traveled back and forth between Southern California and Hawaii, looking like the free-spirited soul with long blond hair and a suntanned body—but that was only the outer image.

By summer's end, I had sold my surfboard and decided to go back to California. Lost and overwhelmed with intense feelings of separation, I had no idea what to do with my life, and neither did my parents. A few months later, a friend joined the U.S. Navy. I had never paid attention to the draft or what military service was really about, but I didn't know what else to do, and it was easier to sign up with Uncle Sam than to look for a job. It was a drastic choice, but I was desperate for a direction.

The night before joining the Navy as a seaman apprentice, I went to a party and got really loaded. My friends and I were driving with booze, pills, and pot in the car and got pulled over by the cops. When we began throwing things out the window, we were arrested and taken to jail. I told the cops I was leaving for boot camp in San Diego the next morning, and they just shook their heads and let me go.

The next day I woke up in a daze from the night before, but somehow made it to the bus that transported us all to boot camp. I slept most of the way from Los Angeles to San Diego, about a two-and-a-half-hour drive. As the bus drove onto the military base, I looked out the window at an alien world. Everyone was wearing uniforms, and they all looked alike. I saw white stucco buildings with red-tiled roofs neatly lined up as far as I could see. When I realized the magnitude of what I had done, fear rose up in me. I thought, "Tom, where are you, and what have you done?"

I got off the bus and joined about 400 guys in line to get our heads shaved. My last haircut had been the one they had made me get in order to return to school in the twelfth grade. A military official looked at me and said, "What are you, one of those L.A. hoods or surfers? Come with me, punk." He put me at the front of the line and I had my head shaved. This shameful walk only confirmed my fears; I realized then that joining the military was a huge mistake.

I made it through boot camp and about a year on the Navy ship to which I was assigned, but I became very fed up with the military lifestyle. After a weekend at home, I decided not to go back to my ship, taking a leave of absence without permission. I hit the streets for about thirty days; no haircuts. I had my ear pierced, and got really wasted.

I still had the problem of the military. I devised a surefire exit strategy. I figured if I returned to the ship but refused to cooperate, the Navy would give me a discharge. I returned late at night as our ship was preparing to leave for another few weeks at sea. This vessel was a huge guided missile cruiser with a brig overseen by Marines. When I went aboard, the officer on duty told me to go to sleep. The next morning, I was taken to the masters-at-arms' office, which operates as a center for the ship's police force.

My plan was to do whatever it took to get off the ship, hoping to be sent to the naval hospital and be declared unfit for the Navy. We were in the middle of San Diego Harbor, pulling out for our big voyage but not yet in open waters. When the masters-at-arms turned their backs on me, I darted away, running through the ship with Marines chasing after me. This pursuit only increased my madness and resolve. I pushed and shoved them as I ran through small passageways, screaming, "Out of my way!"

I finally made it up to the third deck and saw that the ship was moving through the water to the open sea. Marines came up behind me, yelling, "Stop right where you are!"

I ran toward the railing and saw a long drop to the water below. At this point I was on automatic pilot, and there was no turning back. Without hesitation, I flung myself over the railing with all my clothes on, including my heavy cord jacket and desert boots. After hitting the water, it was a struggle to swim with the weight of my clothes; the best I could do was tread water. Finding it hard to claim any victory as I bobbed up and down in the sea, I surrendered and was pulled back aboard by an irritated sailor who had been lowered into the water in a small boat to capture this madman.

I spent five months in all in the Navy brig, but was discharged from the Navy in January of 1966. Amazingly, I was discharged under honorable conditions, with a statement that my mind had become disordered through the use of LSD and other drugs.

While AWOL from the Navy during those thirty days, I met a girl named Laura at a party in Malibu. We spent as much of those thirty days together as we could. She was a senior in high school at the time. She had waited for me and even visited me while I was serving my five months in the Navy brig. I was astounded and moved by her loyalty and affections. After she graduated in June of 1966, we headed for Hawaii. We lived on the North Shore for about three or four months, then headed back to Southern California, where Laura got pregnant. We were married in August of 1966.

Only a few months later we found ourselves fleeing back to Hawaii, with Laura pregnant and my old using buddy Wes tagging along. Upon arrival, we bought a cheap car and headed for the North Shore. Our first two weeks were spent sleeping in parks while looking for a place to live. I smoked dope and took "reds and yellows," which nonaddicts commonly use as sleeping pills. Every night I passed out. Nothing bothered me, including the rain and mosquitoes. I slept great. With the continuous use of drugs, I had mastered this type of nomadic existence.

In September 1967, we found an attractive little two-bedroom house just two houses from the ocean on Ke Nui Road at Sunset Beach, directly in front of a popular surfing spot called Rocky Point. The North Shore was beautiful in the sixties. The beaches were empty, with white sand, picturesque palm trees, and the most perfect waves in the world.

As we began meeting many of the people living on the North Shore, I discovered that LSD and hashish were freely available; so these became my drugs of choice. I embraced the shared experience; it became like communion with psychedelics. I felt good about not shooting dope, convincing myself that part of my life was over. I was happy to be part of the spiritual movement popular with most people in our community. A group of us regularly came together to go into the woods to meditate. We would hike up into the mountains overlooking the coastline, where you could see for miles in either direction. The waves would line up on the horizon as they pushed their way forward to the shore. It was like each wave knew its destiny, finding its way to the coastline of the North Shore near the end of its journey.

We would sit in a circle as someone read a spiritual book guiding us to higher realms of consciousness. We all wore white muslin yoga pants, considered fashionable at the time. Everyone practiced yoga and sat in the lotus position. The lotus position is a popular way to sit when meditating because it keeps your back straight. Keeping the spine erect is important and something always emphasized when learning to meditate. This was a huge problem for me, because ever since childhood, flexibility was not my friend. I couldn't even touch my toes. I couldn't sit in a cross-legged position, let alone in a lotus. This just added to the ever-growing separation I had first experienced in kindergarten. The drugs took away those feelings in the beginning, but not anymore.

There we all were, getting into position on the mountaintop. Since I didn't haul a chair up the mountain with me, I found myself taking a kneeling position to maintain proper positioning.

"Okay," I thought, "I've got it together: positioned properly, yoga pants on, hair is long (I hadn't had a haircut since I was discharged from the Navy almost two years earlier), haven't shaved. God, I'm looking good here."

Then the reading started. Eyes closed, yet looking upward—they say this is where the third eye is, where the light is—I was high on LSD and had also smoked some marijuana. I was totally ready for the journey. About six or seven minutes into the meditation, my legs started to cramp, and I felt the circulation completely cut off.

"Ok, just listen to the prayers being read. You can transcend this feeling of pain," I thought.

More time went on, but all I could hear were my thoughts: "I know I will never be able to walk again. I'm sure my legs are turning purple. I will have to be airlifted off the mountain. I can't take it. I have to move, but then they will all know I'm not in a deep meditation." At that point, though, I didn't care. Slowly, and as quietly as I could, I changed positions. With every quiet bend, my knees would defiantly pop or lock themselves in place. Who knew enlightenment would be so painful? I had to lie down and stretch my legs out before it was too late. I lay on my back and started to extend my legs. The pain was really bad, but I got them straight, lay back, and tried to listen.

I thought, "This feels so good now. I can totally stay in this position as long as this goes on. And, hey, my back is still in a straight position."

"I'm starting to enjoy this now. Whoops, it feels like there is a bug in my pants! Just focus, Tom. Don't move!"

I stayed still, but I had to move again to scratch my butt. Then I had to pick my nose. "Stop it," I shouted to my mind. "Can't you stay focused?"

So there I lay, knowing everyone was in bliss and I was preoccupied with all these bodily sensations, when it hit me....

"God, do I have to pee! There is no way I can hold it much longer, but if I get up to go behind a tree, everyone will know that I'm incapable of meditating for any longer than a few minutes."

As I look back on those days, I can see I was searching for something else. Something in me knew that there was a better life, and I knew meditation was one of the answers, but I couldn't get it. First, I had to stop using. Not only did I not understand that; I didn't know how to stop—yet.

Today I know that everyone is searching for a sense of freedom within, but when our seeking is misdirected, many of us turn to drugs, alcohol, money, relationships, or acquiring more things to fill ourselves. Our spiritual search becomes an endless, and at times terrified, hunt for fulfillment. We label people who abuse drugs and alcohol "addicts," but isn't craving of anything addiction? We fail to realize that all things are impermanent, and that nothing outside of us will ever take away our inner feelings of emptiness and isolation.

On a Sunday at 3:50 p.m., December 24, 1967, my daughter Celeste was born. The small one-story stucco hospital, which was built in the 1920s or 1930s and looked more like plantation housing, was located in Waialua on the North Shore of Oahu. It was nearly empty when we arrived. The doctor and nurse, who were to be in the delivery room with Laura, were the only staff there, and had asked me to watch the office and answer the phone. Were they serious? Of course I would watch the office. Turning an addict loose in a hospital is like releasing a kid in a candy store. I'm not proud to admit it, but while my daughter was being born, I was in the pharmacy stealing syringes and looking for drugs to shoot up. That feeling of being happy I'd had just a few months before was gone. It became too clear that I had no choice about shooting drugs. If I had ever had a choice, it was pushed out of the way as merely a distraction as I frantically searched the cabinets for injectable narcotics. Sadly, in an addict's life, the drugs always come before everything else.

Celeste Noel Catton was a healthy, beautiful baby, and I was a proud father. Her birth was a good thing in my life, a very good thing; but even becoming a father couldn't keep me clean.

Overpowering feelings of separation continued taking over my life, and I had no idea what to do about it. I kept taking drugs in an attempt to find that inner "God consciousness" I had read about in my spiritual books. *Samadhi*, joy, light, and love were what I knew I wanted, but my heart was running on empty. I had been running in place for too long. Despite the confusion and complete chaos in my life, I never forgot that simple line in my SRF lessons: *When the student is ready, the teacher will appear.* I thought maybe I should go to India to search for enlightenment, but the truth was I couldn't even leave the North Shore and go to Honolulu, on the same island, let alone India.

Little did I know, my life was about to change dramatically in a way I never dreamed possible. The miracle was about to take place. The teacher was about to appear.

CHAPTER TWO

THE
MIRACLE

Celeste was now about two months old. I was a full-blown
addict, and quite a far cry from the fatherly Ozzie Nelson on the
popular 1950s TV show "The Adventures of Ozzie and Harriet." I
loved my daughter and was primarily into the "spiritual seeking" part
of my addictive drug use. I wasn't shooting dope (except for the time
I stole the syringes from the hospital) and mostly took lots of LSD
and smoked hash. I was "meditating" and exploring various spiritual
paths and gurus. The spiritual books and meditation lessons I was
receiving in the mail gave no indication that drugs could help anyone
on their spiritual path in any way. I had essentially sanctified my using
by creating a self-invented religion of the time—one that allowed for
"mind-expanding drugs," but considered needle-driven drugs to be
for "true" addicts. Only books written by others in the drug culture

supported this behavior. Deep inside, I knew I had to stop. How many times had I said I would stop, only to pick up again and again? How does one stop this insanity? This inner voice would pose these questions to me in quiet and unguarded moments, but I would silence it with spiritual rationalizations or simply another hit off the joint.

Taking daily walks with my daughter in her little backpack carrier along Ke Nui Road, a small one-lane road with the main highway on one side and the ocean on the other, became a special part of my day. If I had any moments of purity or states of holiness in my life, they were found in these gentle strolls with Celeste. Our daily path was lined with foliage separating us from the busy main road. We would stop and admire the flowers and the tiny bugs that lived amidst the greenery, crawling here and there for us to watch. The earth would seem to come alive and attempt to impress us with this magical matinee. Since I didn't work, I was able to spend every day with my newborn daughter. Yet, as we took our walks viewing the nature around us, the disease would pull me back. I was still feeling separated from the world and its inhabitants and was very paranoid at times. I was unable to experience the "oneness of life" that is promised by following the various spiritual paths I was reading about. I certainly didn't identify with the freedom, love, and peace preached by flower children in the sixties. I was totally lost in the desperation of addiction, but didn't know it. Since I wasn't shooting drugs into my veins or taking pills, I kept trying to convince myself that I was okay. Addiction is most certainly a disease of denial.

Next door to our little two-bedroom home was a four-bedroom beach house that had been vacant for several months. Early one morning a car pulled into the driveway of this house, and I saw a lady get out and go into the house. Later in the day, there was talk in the neighborhood about a strange-looking lady who had moved into the beach house.

The second time I saw this woman, who called herself Flobird, she was standing on the white, sandy beach in front of the house, dressed in a bikini. She had long salt-and-pepper hair that she always wore in a distinctive style—a bun pinned on top and the rest falling to her waist. She was tall and skinny, her face wrinkled and her skin weathered from years in the sun.

As I approached this woman, with the sun beginning to set into the ocean behind her, I felt something I had not felt in so long. We began to talk, and I felt good inside. I didn't feel the anxiety in my stomach that I always carried. She told me she was a beachcomber. "I pick up lost souls and lead them to a spiritual life." Flobird looked directly into my eyes, almost as if she could see through to my soul. I felt so much love from her and knew that she understood me completely—even the pain I carried within. Comfort seemed to emanate from her, and my thoughts seemed to clear away for a wordless message. In that instant, I remembered what I had read in my meditation lesson: *When the student is ready, the teacher will appear.*

I later learned that before finding twelve-step programs and getting into recovery in 1960, Flobird was considered a hopeless type of addict. As a result of decades of addiction to drugs and alcohol, she had seriously abused her body. At one point in her early recovery, she experienced severe physical and emotional problems. A doctor told Flobird that her liver was shot and she was dying. He gave her six months to live.

Nearly everyone who met Flobird could sense this unconditional love radiating from her. Her entire being poured out joy, light, and love. At the time of our meeting, she had about eight years in recovery.

Flobird told me this story:

"A year-and-a-half after coming to the program, I came home from a meeting and the pains had taken over my body. I started getting liver attacks. I called my supervisor where I worked at the time and said I had to quit. Seeking direction, I went to the Bible, as I usually did, closed my eyes, and placed my finger on the page I had opened to. It said: *If you can't leave houses, husbands, children, and wives to follow me, you're not worthy of me.* Then I picked up the twelve-step program book, flipped it open, and put my finger down on a page that said: *We have to be willing to go to any lengths.*

"Then I called my husband, from whom I was separated, and asked if he wanted to get back together. He said no, because he never had it so good. I said that was okay, and that he could have everything—our house in Riverside, California, and all the assets. Walking out the door was the hardest thing I have ever done.

"I ended up at Imperial Beach, just north of the Mexican border. I took my gear and went out on the sand dunes, where I stayed for forty days.

"I was on a beach with hundreds of seagulls and pelicans. In the morning, they'd rise up and fly. The pelicans were so beautiful, and I'd feel lifted up. Several times in my mind I'd think I'd already died and gone to heaven with the birds.

"The pains in my body became unbearable, and my ankles were swelling. One morning, I just lay down and said, 'Okay I'm ready.' I knew I was dying.

"And then the obsession to drink hit me. I looked at the ocean and thought it was vodka. I crawled down to the edge to get a drink and crawled back up. I don't know how long this went on, but as I was lying there, suddenly there was stillness. I mentally saw the universe as pure, vibrating light. I spiritually experienced it.

"All knowledge was open to me. I saw that everything was perfect in its changing form. Most people don't know that. They have to wake up. The vibrations, like 10,000 volts of electricity, went through my body. Love and joy went through me, and I was awake for the first time in my life.

"My body began to heal, and after another two weeks I packed my stuff and walked back into the world. I now knew that my life was no longer mine. I was a channel to give away God's love."

After listening to Flobird's story, I experienced an amazing insight. I knew I had found something I had been looking for all my life. Even though I had no words to describe it, a feeling entered my heart that I wanted what this person had.

From that day on, Flobird considered herself a beachcomber, and the ocean became her beloved friend. In twelve-step meetings, she always talked about the birds: "Look at the birds. They live in the moment, taking no thought for their lives, food, or where they will lay their heads." That's how Florence (her birth name) got the nickname "Flobird."

Flobird gave her life completely to God. She frequently said, "I'm sure of God and He is sure of me." When she walked away from her house in Riverside, she gave up all of her worldly possessions. She asked for nothing from her husband or society; she told us that she totally trusted that "God would provide wherever He guides."

This is how Flobird entered my life that eventful morning in 1968. She had been living and helping out at a recovery halfway house for alcoholics and addicts in Kaneohe, which was about forty miles from the North Shore of Oahu. That morning, as usual, she had been meditating and writing in her journal. Faith can be a conditional thing, but by now Flobird had learned that if she surrendered fully, the direction would come. She was told to go to the North Shore, where she was spiritually guided to the vacant, fully furnished four-bedroom house on the beach. She reached above the door and found the key.

Daring to follow her heart, Flobird moved in. When the realtor arrived the next day to show the house, he discovered Flobird and asked what she was doing there. "God told me to come here," she said. "Can you please have the electricity turned on?"

Needless to say, it was turned on, and Flobird lived in this house for about six months. This was my introduction to the modern-day miracle, an event that was to become a common experience over the next ten years that Flobird was in my life.

When I met her I was incredibly lost in the world of addiction. The using and despair had left me on autopilot, traveling in circles. But I was also seeking a better way of life by learning how to meditate and become more spiritual. The deep feelings of separation, fear of life, and complete emptiness were so strong inside of me. All I could do was take more drugs in an attempt to fill an emptiness that couldn't be filled by anything outside of me. No amount of drugs, my wife, a baby, money, sex—nothing worked. The despair and the feeling that I didn't belong anywhere now dominated all of my thoughts and actions.

My talks with Flobird were the first time I had ever heard anything said about a twelve-step recovery program. It was difficult for me to understand her because I had never thought of myself as an addict. After all, everyone I hung out with used alcohol and drugs the way I did. Our ever-present misery just seemed to be another facet of the lifestyle, almost like a tattoo that symbolizes what gang or tribe you belong to.

In February 1968, Flobird started one of the first twelve-step meetings on the North Shore. It was held at the beach house and attended mostly by recovering addicts from Honolulu. I was about to take another step on my journey of self-discovery.

I was afraid to go to the first meeting, but I did walk back and forth on the tree-covered lane to and from the beach, gazing into Flobird's living room window each time I walked by. I was unable to walk into a house full of people I didn't know. Even people I *did* know would have been too scary. Fear dominated my life.

Somehow, I made it to the second meeting at the beach house. I heard people say they felt at home at their first twelve-step meeting because they had heard others talk openly about how obsessively they drank and used drugs. They identified with those stories and came back. That wasn't what brought me back. At my first meeting, someone talked about feeling like a misfit in a world where everyone else had it all together. This was the first time I had ever heard anyone verbalize feelings of separation, the same feelings that had been an overwhelming part of my life since that day I was dropped off at kindergarten. I had never heard those words spoken. I had never heard another verbalize and make that pain, and its underlying fear, real. I was finally beginning to wake up from the bad dream.

Never before had I heard people talk so honestly about their feelings. It was entirely new for me to be with a group of people who openly shared their innermost emotions. Once I was able to start sharing, I experienced a great sense of relief. Any initial awkwardness was soon swept away by the understanding and love of the other addicts I had found sitting in that circle. It was my first experience of the miracle that takes place when we express what is inside of us. I found out early on that if I shared my pains and fears at a meeting, they were lessened by the time I left; and if I shared the joy and fulfillment I felt, I'd have more of it when I left. It's called a giveaway program.

So, the miracle began the day Flobird appeared and when I began attending meetings. I realized I was an addict and the Twelve Steps *could* be *my* spiritual path. Although I didn't stay clean from my first meeting, a spark of hope had entered my heart. Something strongly told me to fan that flame, to guard this precious gift. This was the beginning of a three-year journey that would eventually take me to my bottom, a place of overwhelming hopelessness that all addicts must visit in order to be open to receive the gift of willingness in our lives.

CHAPTER THREE

THE GIFT

The next three years proved to be a true initiation leading me to my spiritual path. Following this course required a deep surrender of my life. I had to get out of my own way so grace could penetrate my deep-rooted walls of denial. This required committed spiritual practice, at times, through enormous upheavals in my life. Hitting bottom on drugs was my gift; this painful experience was what it took for me to begin the awakening of my spirit within.

When we find ourselves in deep pain or crisis situations, we can be led in a new direction. It's like walking through a door and discovering that all we thought familiar has fallen away. Then the way we perceive life changes profoundly. Life and its many changes can be a movement toward the Divine.

After six months in that North Shore beach house, which became known has the "God house," Flobird once again received direct guidance from her Higher Power during meditation. These messages often came in the form of "Prepare to leave this place," sometimes even indicating where she should go. Other directives told her to "Pack up your stuff and walk out the door." This time she was told, "Head for Maui."

During those six months, I went to a lot of meetings and let go of much denial about my addiction, but I still couldn't stop using drugs. I would stay clean for a few weeks, only to find myself picking up drugs again. Some of my fellow drug users came to the meetings, understood the message, and stopped using. I was baffled as to why I kept picking up. I was hearing this message of recovery with an open mind, but I began to feel I was too open, and the message would slip right through me. I would find myself loaded yet again.

Although I couldn't stop using, living around Flobird and going to the meetings at her house was starting to enrich my inner feelings. Hope, something I wasn't familiar with, started to bubble up within. After Flobird left, everything seemed empty again on the North Shore. So, after finding some friends to watch our house, Laura and I, along with our now nine-month-old daughter Celeste and our two German shepherds, boarded a plane headed for Maui to find Flobird. I had learned this much in my short time with Flobird: The spiritual search calls for willing seekers to take that crucial next step. We traveled with faith and trust pushing us onward.

We knew from her letters that she was living in the then-largely unpopulated area of Makena Beach. We started hitchhiking. The beauty of the area was breathtaking. There were many kiawe trees on this dry side of the island, and their huge green thorns appeared stunning against the blue sky and vast ocean. It took a while, but we eventually found Flobird living about five miles down a dirt road that ran along spectacular white sand beaches that seemed to stretch forever. Her home was a huge white house located right on the ocean, with only a few close neighbors. Ironically, several hundred feet away was a home occupied by Timothy Leary, who had played such a huge part in my early drug-using days. There I was with Flobird living in a house representing recovery, and Leary turning on and tuning out at a nearby house representing the ugly, addictive part of my life. The irony was remarkable, and I was mindful that it was like standing at one of the many crossroads of life.

Every morning I watched Flobird as she sat in front of her house, facing the ocean and meditating. Across the way, Leary also sat on his deck looking at the ocean, probably tripping on acid, since this was the path he presented to the world. As I watched, it almost looked like a standoff on the spiritual path.

Living in this house right on the ocean proved to be a time to deepen my understanding of the twelve-step programs. We were pretty isolated, being five miles down a dirt road, so I was able to stay clean the whole time. We had impromptu meetings most days, and I would never tire of listening to Flobird talk about the spiritual life. It seemed I didn't have to even understand or grasp intellectually everything she talked about. It was as though her heart was talking to my heart. Something was deepening within me.

It was hot and sunny each day, and we would spend time on the beach swimming and playing. When dawn started to come upon us, I would find myself sitting on the front deck each morning. I was learning the discipline of being quiet. Doing a meditation before the day started was like greeting the day as it gave birth to the light. Each evening we would find ourselves on the deck again as the sun set behind a cloudless horizon. I would even find myself saying good-bye to the sun and thanking it for the beautiful day. This goodness within that I had felt the first time I met Flobird was starting to expand as each day passed.

After being on Maui for about a month, Laura and I returned to our North Shore house, but it began to feel uncomfortable, as if our time there had come to an end. So we started selling our things and gathering money to leave Hawaii and head back to California.

We found a nice little cottage to rent that was set behind a homeowner's main house in Venice. The backyard was full of trees and plants, with an enormous pine tree right at the front entrance of our new house. It seemed almost like an isolated country home. It was a pleasant transition into the city from rural Hawaii. I got my hair cut and tried working a bit.

Laura got pregnant again, and I tried living a somewhat normal type of life, although my drug using continued. I felt I had enough understanding of recovery to monitor and stay on top of the using, thinking I could run on the fumes of what I had gathered being around Flobird. We stayed in touch with Flobird, and I even went to some twelve-step meetings while in California. I now knew I had the disease of addiction, but just could not seem to find a way to surrender.

Flobird had received guidance to leave Hawaii and stayed in our area for a week or so before heading to the East Coast. It was great to see her again, and I even managed to get a little clean time going. My friend Ronnie, the surfing and drug-using buddy who previously lived next door to me, came over and met Flobird. Like nearly everyone she met, his heart was touched, and he eventually got clean. He now has nearly thirty years in recovery. We continued to receive letters from Flobird, who ended up staying in Virginia Beach for a couple of months before heading back to Hawaii.

Later that year, another good friend, Tom M., had just been released from Atascadero Mental Institution for the Criminally Insane. We had used drugs together since the early 1960s, and I had always judged his addiction as much worse than mine. I used him as a dark measure of my own using and life, and tried to convince myself that I would never get that bad or go that far. He came over and we began smoking pot and getting high. He said he wanted to go to Hawaii, so I told him about the islands and Flobird (who was now living back in Hawaii), and the twelve-step programs she had introduced me to. In a sense, I was carrying the message of recovery to Tom. Since I was getting high with him, I don't think I was very coherent, but nevertheless, it was my first "twelve-step call."

At the time, Tom could barely talk. He stuttered terribly, and the behavior that resulted from his drug use almost made him seem less than human. I wanted to help him, so I told him, "The North Shore of Oahu is the place to go because all the young people are out there." I also showed him a photo of Flobird and described her as an "alcoholic and addict," which was strange because I certainly never used those words before my introduction to twelve-step meetings. In the hopeless circles I ran in, those words were never part of our vocabulary. Tom later told me that he interpreted my murky message as "There's this weird woman, and if you get hard up you could shack up with an old alkie."

Within a few weeks, Tom was off to Hawaii. He landed at the airport in Honolulu around 10 p.m. and began hitchhiking out to the North Shore, which is about forty-five miles away. He soon realized that Hawaii wasn't a small island that you could ride your bicycle around. There were no grass shacks to sleep in. No beautiful Hawaiian ladies in grass skirts were welcoming him. He was greeted with the indifference of an empty moonlit highway.

Tom was dropped off at Sunset Beach, one of the many big-wave surfing spots, at about 1 a.m. He wandered down to the beach and fell asleep under the thick bushes and palm trees. When Tom awakened in the morning, reality set in. He had traveled to Hawaii, where he knew no one and had no money to buy dope. He realized he had made a huge mistake. He had found himself alone, broke, and strung out in paradise.

Sitting alone on the beach, Tom felt totally desperate and confused. Flobird, who was living in a house about a half-mile up the beach, was practicing her daily two-hour routine of early-morning meditation, writing in her journal, and waiting for specific guidance about how she was to live the rest of her day. She later told us that all of a sudden, she received this message: "Go to Sunset Beach NOW!"

Coming out of her bedroom, Flobird woke up several recovering addicts who were then living with her, the same guys I had hung out with when I first met her.

"Get the car started, I have to get to the beach," she told them.

"Can't you just walk across the street to the beach?" they asked.

"No," said Flobird, her voice filled with urgency. "I have to get to Sunset Beach right now!"

Flobird drove a short distance down the highway and pulled up to Sunset Beach. She got out of her car, walked down to the ocean's edge, and put her hands on her hips.

"Okay, God. Here I am. What's up?"

Tom was what was up, crawling out from under the bushes in a state of extreme confusion. He looked up and saw the lady in the photo I had shown to him in California. He staggered toward her and began mumbling. She could not understand him, but said, "You are why I'm here. Put your stuff in my car." It was December 17, 1968; Tom has been in recovery since that day.

I have since learned there are no coincidences in life. But there are miracles we can all experience and connect with when we are fully awake, mindful of life in the moment, and unafraid to follow our hearts. They only ask of us our presence, an acknowledgment, and our attention paid in full. Love merely generates more of itself, with little or no notice.

I soon began getting letters from Tom. I couldn't believe it. Even in his letters, the miracle in his life was apparent. There had obviously been a colossal change, because he was no longer the same confused person I last saw in California. He had come fully alive. His spirit was awakening. It could be felt on the pages of the letter.

But there I was, still using. It seemed to me that all the addicts who ran into Flobird were getting clean and staying that way. What was going on with me? Why was I immune to this magic? Had I somehow left the room during the big initiation? Since the day I met Flobird, had gone to my first meeting, and found out I had this disease, I wanted to stop. But I was caught in the insanity, the compulsion to use, and nothing seemed to relieve this for any real length of time. As I look back, I can see it was not time for me to answer my invitation to walk through the door of grace. I was not done—not ready within.

Our son, Joshua Bird, was born on September 4, 1969, and we headed back to the Sunset Beach area of Hawaii right after Christmas. We stayed with friends until we found a house across the street from a beach called Sharks Cove. I began going to meetings once again and staying clean for short periods. When Flobird was in town, we had meetings at my house, but after everyone left, I got loaded. It seemed like my resolve was strong when I was safely encircled with other clean addicts, but that determination would leave with them when we said our good-byes. I truly didn't want to use, but I was powerless over the obsession to use drugs. During 1970 I actually stayed clean twice, for more than three months each time.

Flobird and a bunch of her followers lived in tents across the street in the grassy park overlooking Sharks Cove. By now there were several people who had met Flobird, started going to meetings, and weren't using drugs or alcohol anymore. They were a bunch of spiritual nomads, helping one another stay clean as they tried to help others who were ready to surrender. She was like a shepherd with a willing flock of misfits, all of them miracles, all of them clean. Then one morning she awoke at an early hour and was given this message: "Go to Egypt by boat." After she announced this to us, preparations began for the adventure. Since I was married and had two kids, I certainly wasn't going to join them, and neither was the other Tom. Flobird and her group left for their new journey.

One evening toward the end of the year, I smoked a joint and drank two beers in a friend's tent. At the time, I had over three months clean. I went into convulsions on the tent floor, and after coming out of it, I said, "Wow, I'm allergic to this stuff." I didn't get loaded for a few days, but even after drugs and alcohol had demonstrated monstrous effects on me physically, I still began using again. We flew to California for Christmas in 1970, and once again, I began using more heavily.

I had heard in meetings how the disease can progress even when we aren't using. Now I was experiencing it in my life, and I was quickly spiraling to my bottom. When we returned to Hawaii, the needles came out and I became strung out again. For the next ten months, I shot dope constantly. It almost killed me.

I was shooting coke and heroin every day. My arms became tattooed with bruises, track marks, and lesions. It got to the point that when I went to score drugs, the dealers didn't want me to use there. "Just get the drugs and leave," they said. I had become so hopeless that other addicts didn't want me around. They ran me off, fearing I might contaminate their scene. I wandered around the North Shore in my swim trunks, carrying a syringe in an envelope in my shorts. I used garden hoses from private homes to get water to dissolve the dope, and shot up in the bushes. I would be missing for days at a time and then wander into my house. Naturally, my wife was fed up with this behavior.

When I couldn't score dope, I shot caffeine or wine into my veins, causing an instant hangover. I was once more guided by desperation, traveling again in terror. I frequently woke up on the beach under a palm tree with my face planted in the sand. There was no difference between me and a homeless person on skid row. I had arrived at that place where skid row was within, and it didn't matter if I was sleeping in a dumpster, in some dark alley, or on a beautiful beach. Skid row was the constant feelings of hopelessness and despair in my heart. Skid row is in the mind of the hopeless. These feelings were, perhaps, magnified because I had been introduced to a different way of life by Flobird, but I still couldn't get it. What she taught seemed just out of my grasp, so like a good dope fiend, I reached for the painfully familiar. I had resigned myself to a downhill ride.

Laura finally had an "enlightened experience" and decided to leave me. As I look back, I wonder why it took her so long. Then, something unexplainable happened. We talked about her leaving, and I begged her to leave Josh, now nearly two years old, with me. She would take Celeste back to California with her. Seeing my grief and desperation, with compassion as her guide she agreed to leave Josh in my care, and somehow knew on a deep level he would be cared for. In hindsight, I see that it was all part of a divine plan. I really believe Josh was what kept me alive. I now can identify with the single mom burdened with addiction.

I'm not proud about what happened over the next couple of months. Even now, it's difficult to write about this period without crying. I never had a clean and sober moment from the time Laura left in early August. I stayed stoned all that time, hitchhiking around the area with Josh to score dope. I went to parties on the beach, left him in someone's parked car, and proceeded to get stoned.

One night around midnight, I had run out of dope. I knew someone in Ewa Beach who had some drugs, so at 1 a.m. I woke my son and we walked out to the darkened highway, lit only by the headlights of passing cars, fueled by the relentless obsession that burned through my body and numbed my thinking. We hitchhiked across the island, a distance of some fifty miles from the North Shore. I scored, shot up, and started hitchhiking back home with my drugs. This is the insanity of the addict. At times, I left Josh at home with friends who had moved in after Laura left. The next morning, I couldn't even remember how I got home.

I was so caught up in the obsession to use drugs that I couldn't do anything but continue using. One day while caring for Josh, I was changing his diaper. He was lying on his back on the bed crying. Somehow in this moment, just my precious baby boy and me, I really heard him and saw him. I had a moment of clarity. I felt and I knew then, deep inside my gut, I had to get Josh back to his mother.

A few days later, on October 20, 1971, I woke up. I had heroin, pot, hashish, and lots of pills and alcohol in the house. My normal response would be to wake up, run and puke in the toilet or over the back porch, and proceed to get stoned.

I was feeling especially hopeless that morning. Flobird was in Egypt with her followers. Tom M., who was on Maui, called me at least once a week to see if I was alive. I would cry on the phone, telling him I wanted to stop using drugs but couldn't. I couldn't stop using, and I couldn't even get high.

For some reason, I didn't get high the minute I woke up. Instead, I took Josh and walked across the street to Sharks Cove. I sat on the cliff, looking down at the lava rocks. It was gray and gloomy, and the ocean was unusually stormy. I began to cry uncontrollably. Tears streamed down my face, and Josh started crying. At that moment, I experienced a feeling of total powerlessness. All the years of denial just flew out of me. I was dead but still walking around. I knew there was no hope of my ever changing.

I cried out to God, "If you are real, I need help now."

Something happened that morning to expedite my spiritual journey that I'm still only coming to fully understand. All of a sudden, it was as though someone had wrapped a warm blanket around me and was gently holding me. A tremendous feeling of peace coursed through my body. It was the first time I had ever experienced such peace and stillness.

In that moment, I felt nearly whole and complete. I heard a voice say, "You never have to use again." I sat there in awe, knowing that something powerful had just happened to me.

I picked Josh up and headed back to the house. I packed up some clothes and told my roommates I had to get to Maui and find Tom M. They later told me that they knew something profound had happened to me. I had no money but had been making candles that I planned to sell for drug money. I grabbed a large candle in the shape of a mushroom, and Josh and I walked out to the highway to hitchhike to the airport. I felt a new sense of calm, yet moved decisively, trusting this awakened intuition.

I tried to sell the candle to each driver who stopped for us, but no one seemed interested. Still, I continued on to the airport, with this powerful drive within me knowing I would get to Maui. When we got to the airport, I still hadn't sold the candle. I had no money but got in a line of about ten people anyway to buy our plane ticket. By the time I got to the counter, I had sold the candle for the exact amount of the plane fare. This experience of being provided for in a moment of great need would be repeated many times in the years to come.

After landing on Maui, we hitchhiked to Lahaina. I didn't know where Tom M. lived, just that he was in the Lahaina area. As our ride pulled into the town, I looked up and saw one of Tom's brothers standing on the street. I got out of the car and said, "Where's Tom?" He directed me to a house up the street. I walked in and said, "I'm ready to do anything to stay clean."

Tom later said he also saw something different in me, an ease in my presence, a lightening of my shadow. We went to a meeting that night; and after a few days of going to meetings on Maui, I returned to the North Shore.

I also knew something overpowering and life-changing had happened to me that morning at Sharks Cove. I had been given a great gift and decided to do everything I could to hang onto it. I had been using heavily for the previous ten months, shooting up anything I could get into a syringe. But now, coming off drugs, I experienced no withdrawal symptoms at all. This was unheard of for any dope fiend of my category, and I realized that God was protecting me as if I wore some invisible amulet. I no longer questioned this precious gift. I acknowledged it in my life and moved forward.

I began borrowing cars, hitchhiking, and doing whatever I could to get to meetings. The gift of willingness was given to me, and today, thirty-nine years later, I still have that same willingness to go to any lengths to stay clean. It has been my direction and message to others. Whenever I share my story at a twelve-step meeting or a convention, this is always an important part of my message of recovery—the willingness to do anything it takes to stay clean.

Since that day, October 20, 1971, the obsession to use has never returned. I know in my heart that there was and is a spiritual force working in my life. In that one decisive moment on the beach, I was transformed. Having been released from active addiction, I now know that no matter what, life is for me and not against me. I have come out the other side of my addiction as a better person. I realize that life has many obstacles, but walking through them clean and sober only brings me closer to an inner place of love and joy—to a connection with a power greater than myself. What I mistook for terror were simply signs I may have misunderstood. It was all part of an esoteric initiation, and once I became willing, the universe seemed to carry me along.

After returning to the North Shore, I knew it was time to take Josh back to his mother. So I began preparing to leave Hawaii, packing up and selling what little I had. I started making amends to those around me. I paid back some money I owed, and I bought our plane tickets. On November 8, Josh and I left the Islands. I had less than $100 on me when I landed in California. And so the rest of my journey began.

CHAPTER FOUR

THE JOURNEY BEGINS

When Flobird would receive guidance, one of her favorite sayings was "On we go with the cosmic show!" She understood that she was an instrument and would be guided to her next assignment. She always did this without any thought for her life. She rarely questioned it, and even if she did, she always walked into the unknown. These were the lessons I was beginning to learn. I was developing an inner understanding of hope, faith, belief, and trust, with Flobird leading by example.

I began to see that what I called "my life," in fact, really wasn't. I was beginning to see how I had been operating under the illusion of self-seeking ego, and that delusion only fed my feelings of separateness. To find true fulfillment, I would have to be willing to give of myself. From the very beginning, Flobird taught me to strive to become a channel to be used for service to others. She made it clear in the way she lived her life, and I desperately wanted to live that way.

"Let God, the universe—or whatever you choose to call it—know it is okay to use you to help others get clean and to carry this message. The message is the spiritual awakening. Allow it to become your life's work," Flobird said. "Put that work ahead of everything else, knowing that God will take care of the rest of your life on a daily basis."

Looking back, I can truly say this has happened; it is still happening.

When Josh and I landed at the airport in Los Angeles, it was a cold winter day. Laura and Celeste picked us up. They both looked so beautiful dressed in their warm winter clothes. Celeste was almost four years old. She wore an orange-yellow corduroy jumpsuit with a matching jacket. Laura wore a wool sweater and jeans and boots. Her brown hair seemed a bit longer, and she appeared to have a certain glow about her. I felt so much love upon seeing her. Josh clung to me, a bit hesitant to be held right away in his mother's arms. The transition took a while, but he soon seemed at home with his mother and sister.

Taking Josh back to his mother and sister was so right, so beautiful. Of course, all of us being together again made me wonder why I couldn't also be part of that family. There were many painful moments in those first few months. Although I still had feelings for Laura, I also saw how my addiction had destroyed so much of the trust we once had. These were hard realizations to accept, but I did my best, and most importantly, I didn't use.

The same was true with my parents, who were happy I was not using, yet were understandably hesitant to lower their guard with me. I knew this time was different, but it would take a while for the people close to me who had been hurt so many times by my addictive behavior to see that my recovery was real.

I started going to meetings right away and connected with others in the recovery community. I would find places to sleep each night, bouncing around from my parents to Laura and to the many people I had met in meetings who opened their doors and couches to me. I took the suggestions that were freely given and did my best to live the life of recovery. Now that I was on the mainland living in California, my goal was to find Flobird and her group in Egypt. I needed money to travel, so I began making candles like I had been doing in Hawaii. It was November and I knew Christmas would be a good time to sell them.

A lady named Evelyn, whom I met in the program, let me use her garage to set up my little candle-making factory. So I started making candles during the day, and at night, after twelve-step meetings, I went to the garage to fire up the burners and melt the different colors of wax. I focused on creating mushroom-shaped candles in a variety of sizes, using cups and bowls for molds, and then a torch to melt recessed areas on the top part of the candle, which created an uneven surface. As I melted the top surface of the wax, the colors from beneath would shine through with the light reflecting.

The California nights were cold compared to winter nights in Hawaii. The garage would heat up a bit as the wax melted. My radio was tuned to my favorite pop stations during these late nights. The music not only came from the radio, but also seemed to be coming from my heart. It would fill me with an inner joy. I didn't realize it at the time, but my spirit within was waking up.

I was clean and feeling good. Life seemed so simple, and I was joyful much of the time. Members of twelve-step programs call it the "honeymoon period" of early recovery. I was "high" off not getting high. During this time, I was invited to give a ten-minute speech at a huge meeting in the Los Angeles area, usually attended by several hundred people. "It's so good to be clean, and I never have to hurt again," I told the group. That got a big laugh from the audience because they knew the truth: Get the drugs and alcohol out of the way, and pretty soon you have to start dealing with all the emotional baggage inside, which doesn't always feel good.

This was my first Christmas and New Year in recovery. The red and green of the seasonal lights seemed a little crisper, and the familiar caroling was more inviting to my ears. The spirit of Christmas was in my newly awakened heart. I went to a party hosted by one of the twelve-step groups. I was nervous about trying to dance without being loaded on some sort of chemical. But then it happened—it was the music again. It flowed through me like a wave of inspiration. Something inside me woke up, and without a second thought I found myself on the dance floor. I discovered I could really have fun being clean. What a gift!

On January 29, 1972, with only a little over three months clean, I'd made enough money selling candles and boarded a plane in L.A. headed for London, en route to Egypt. I was to take a train from London to the bottom tip of Italy, then cross over by ferry to Alexandria, Egypt. Usually, travelers cross through Morocco and head across through Algeria, but rumor had it that people like me with long hair and a beard were hassled on that route, so I avoided that plan.

Landing in London early in the evening, I found the night air was colder than it was in L.A. when I left. The air was damp with fog. The chill seemed to collect in my bones as I looked up and down the street at my alien surroundings. Reality began to set in. The anticipation of my adventure before leaving California was much greater and perhaps a little more romantic than what I was feeling now. Confusion and a bit of fear started to take over. I did my best to let go of these feelings and get into a solution. I looked within to find a peace to know that I wasn't brought this far to be abandoned under some British streetlight. I had found out where a meeting would be on the night I arrived, so without any arrangements for a place to stay, I found my way to the meeting. Walking into the large hall, I saw a gathering of people at the front of the room. Chairs were set up in rows, which is a familiar sight in a meeting place. Even halfway around the world, the act of entering the meeting made me feel as if I were at home. I walked up and introduced myself, letting my fellow members know I had just arrived from the United States. Knowing I didn't have a place to stay, I was hoping someone would offer to take me home after the meeting, maybe even a nice young lady with a distinctive accent; but that didn't happen.

When the meeting ended, it was getting late, and I knew I had to find somewhere to stay. As I walked down the street, I stopped someone who looked about my age and asked where I might find an inexpensive room for the night. I explained I would be taking a train to Italy the next day.

"Come on home to my flat," he said.

We hopped aboard a double-decker bus that transported us to his place. I entered his small apartment on the second floor of an old brick building. He had a couple of roommates and introduced me. I was tired and feeling out of place in this foreign country. An overstuffed, threadbare couch sat in the main room, and he offered that to me as my bed for the night. I was just grateful to be out of the cold.

I slept well but awoke feeling alone. The quiet flat and the reality of my situation only magnified my growing doubts. I wanted to go back to California, but was scared to tell anybody the truth. After all, who was there to tell? Admitting I felt homesick for the familiarity of the life I left behind created a feeling of shame that I wasn't this free-spirited, gypsy traveler. Nevertheless, I forged on with the goal of finding Flobird. I did my best to tune out the nagging fears that followed so closely behind. I found my way to the ferry that traveled to France. I bought some warm English tea and found a seat by a window. Here I was on a ferry between London and France. The famed cliffs of Dover gradually receded as the ferry lurched forward. The ocean was gray and choppy from the strong winds, and cold, salty air blew onto the deck. It certainly didn't look like the blue, warm, glassy Pacific Ocean that I was used to. I told myself I was on an adventure, and there was no turning back, but thoughts of doing so plagued me.

Landing on the other side of the channel in Calais, I hopped on an overnight train to Rome, where I bought donuts and more tea. I peered out the window, gazing with wonder upon the scenery of snow-covered mountains. It was a very different environment for an island guy like me, but beautiful in its own way. As I gazed out the window, my thoughts once again wandered back to California, where I had felt so secure during my first three months in the program. I was cautious of my new surroundings, but also marveled at how far I had come in such a short time. I thought intensely about Laura, Celeste, and Joshua. I tried to cover up the painful feelings of emptiness with fantasies of getting back together with Laura. Of course, that only made me miss her more. I have since learned that it never works to project out of the moment, because there is no reality to this process. We are not meant to be time travelers. It is only by embracing my feelings in this moment, and sharing them with others, that I find peace.

The train pulled into the Rome station. The crowds were intense, with people pushing and shoving and speaking a different language. It took a while for my senses to adjust to all this new information, and I fought the sense of being overwhelmed by the animated scene that surrounded me. It was difficult for me to maneuver my way around. I finally found a cab and asked to be taken to a reasonably priced hotel.

As the cab pulled out into the traffic flow, it was more like getting on a ride at an amusement park, as the driver weaved in and out of traffic with his hand constantly on the horn. I thought, "There must not be any rules on the roadways here except blow your horn loud and long."

As we sped through the streets of Rome, when my hands weren't covering my eyes out of complete fear of an accident at any moment, I noticed the beautiful city. The buildings and architecture were breathtaking. Each intersection had a new design, a statue of some naked figure, and fountains everywhere, with water spouting upward into the blue sky. The marble gods and goddesses seemed ready to come alive at any moment. I was hoping maybe they would direct the frantic scramble of traffic.

Finally, after several near collisions, we arrived at the hotel. I literally fell out of the cab, thanking the driver, more for the fact I was still alive than for the ride. As I paid him the fare, he nodded a brief goodbye and careened back into the insane roadway. The hotel was a three-story building with a wide-open entrance into a courtyard. In the middle of the yard was, of course, a fountain, with benches dispersed around quaint and beautiful gardens. After checking in to my room, I set out to find a travel agency to arrange the rest of my trip. Now that I had made it to Rome, my plan was to get to the southern tip of Italy and then cross over to Egypt by ferry.

The travel agent explained that ferryboats run sporadically during the winter when the sea is rough, and it would be at least a month until one was going to leave again. I walked out of the agency and looked around the looming Roman streets feeling empty, perplexed, homesick, alone, and scared. Exhausted, I felt like a ghost as I shuffled along the street.

I wandered around town in a sort of daze upon discovering my journey had met an obstacle. I had a bite to eat, some pizza. Maybe it was my despairing mood, but it didn't taste that good. Was the crust too thin or too thick? Was the cheese bitter? I'm not sure; I just knew pizza tasted better in California, but from my point of view, life tasted better there too. However, I did visit the Coliseum, sat on the Spanish Steps, and thought, "What now?"

I began talking to some young travelers sitting nearby. Since I had learned to share my feelings in meetings, I admitted to one young man I was confused and didn't know what to do next. He pulled out some drugs from his pocket and said, "Here, this will make you feel better." Of course, that scared the hell out of me, and I rushed back to my hotel. I knew I had to return home to Los Angeles because I missed my kids and the people I had connected with there.

A week before I left for London, I had given all my candle-making equipment to a recovery house for youths in trouble. For weeks, I had been talking in meetings about my planned trip to Egypt, and how it would be months until I returned. I proudly announced I was off on an adventure to find my sponsor and the people traveling with her.

But I painfully discovered that I wasn't an experienced traveler— more like a naïve drifter. I was scared, felt lost, and needed to swallow my pride and be humble enough to leave Europe and admit I had made a mistake. I had only a few months in recovery and I sensed that this was not a good situation to be in, so I booked a ticket to return to California. It seemed like a much safer place for me. My heart lightened as I traveled home, and I was reminded that it was alright to be wrong and to not know all the answers. This was the same earnest humility and powerlessness that got me clean and led me to surrender. I was starting to see that every experience in recovery was in fact a lesson, and I was seeing how each day clean helped me want to stay clean the next day. I was gradually learning that the universe is a kind and loving teacher, always instructing me and at times giving me the answer inside the question. I need only ask. This experience was one of my first lessons in learning to live in the present. When in Europe, all I could think about was being back home in California. Once I returned to California, all I could think about was being in Europe. I realized I had always lived my life that way, never being present, going somewhere and then wanting to be back where I was previously. That cycle never ends when we live out of the moment. We never feel complete inside, because we are always thinking: "If I were somewhere else, then I would be okay." But as we keep reaching outside of ourselves in a futile attempt to end the inner emptiness, we lose our way. This trip taught me a valuable lesson. I began to realize that my Higher Power was only found in the present moment, that *now* was all there was.

When I landed at the L.A. airport I wanted to kiss the ground, although now I had to go back to meetings as the prodigal son with no mansion on the hill awaiting me. This was humiliating, since I had told everyone I would be gone for months, and here I was back again in a week. Actually, I was the only one who beat myself up. I was welcomed back with open arms. Not one person said a negative thing about my one-week trip abroad. People in the program, especially those new to recovery, could identify with my struggle because they had the same fears. Most importantly, I had stayed clean through it all. I started to sense that my self-obsession and self-consciousness were never to my benefit.

I bought a van, fixed it up to live in, found a job as a carpenter, and settled in for a while. I went to lots of meetings, became fascinated with a variety of women, and just lived my life.

I knew I needed guidance from a sponsor. This is someone who helps you in the program, guides you through the steps, someone to go to when you're confused. You can call your sponsor daily if need be, and since Flobird was halfway around the world, I asked a guy, Brandon, who had many years of recovery, to be my sponsor. He was a mellow, peaceful person, and it was obvious there was a Higher Power working in his life. People in recovery need someone to open up to and help them work the Twelve Steps of the program. We cannot do it alone. Once an addict can come to this simple realization and basic admission, countless miracles occur.

I will never forget the first time he really helped me. I would often go over to my soon-to-be-ex-wife's house and visit our kids or babysit while she went out on a date. On this particular night, she came home and said this guy had given her some cocaine. I asked to see it. She unwrapped a tinfoil package, and there it was—the familiar white powder. The disease of addiction came alive, clicking its teeth in my ear.

Immediately, I wanted it. I quickly left and went to Brandon's house. When I told him what had happened, he just smiled and said, "Of course you wanted it, Tom. You're an addict, and this is the most normal reaction you could have had." Somehow, just by telling him about it and listening to his simple reply, peace came back into my life. I began to realize an important facet of the first of the Twelve Steps, one that my very survival depended on: If I ever thought for an instant I could control my using, I would find myself getting loaded and trying to prove that lethal point to myself. By racing from that house and talking with my sponsor, another addict in recovery, I was showing myself I had no control over drugs.

To this day, with thirty-nine years clean, I think I would react the same way. This is still a humbling thing in my life and a knowledge that is a gift. Working in the construction field throughout my recovery, I have seen guys lifting heavy objects, with the veins popping on their arms, and my first thought is how easy it would be for me to give this guy a fix. When going to the doctor and having blood drawn, I always want to grab the needle and do it myself. I have grown to understand I'm an addict and always will be. I have a reprieve—one day at a time—from this deadly disease, contingent on my practicing a spiritual way of life.

To me, this aspect of the program is a blessing. We either live the spiritual principles of the Twelve Steps or we die. We have to keep working on ourselves; there's no kicking back and thinking we have graduated or done enough. I still work the steps and practice the principles of the program, probably even more than I did when I was a newcomer. I remember being at a meeting during my first few months of recovery and hearing a lady say she had fourteen years clean because she continued to not use drugs even when not using made no sense to her. These eventful times come for all of us; and when they do, we must fall back on our willingness to do anything it takes to stay clean. The desperation that originally brought me to my knees has now become a precious gift that keeps me on my feet.

Springtime came to L.A., and I had been back from my overseas adventure for about two months. I was living in my van, going to meetings just about every day, and visiting the Yogananda's center at the Self-Realization Temple. I meditated every morning in my van, and I read every spiritual book that came my way. More and more, I was coming to my own understanding of the Twelve Steps, and my sense of God-consciousness only deepened with my recovery. It was a subtle dance between what I was learning in meetings and what I was discovering in my personal spiritual quest, and I began to notice the similarities between these two sources.

I liked living in my van. Most nights, I parked in a parking lot at Sunset and the Coast Highway. I would back up to the edge of the lot, overlooking the water. Living on the ocean for free, all night I would hear the waves and the water splashing up against the rocks on the shoreline. The sound lulled me to sleep. Life was good.

Someone in the program who had a boat at the marina gave me a key to the restrooms, which had showers for people who lived on their boats. I had access to showers after work each day.

It was the end of March, and I had been in recovery since October. I lived a life of almost monastic simplicity, and began experiencing more and more of the precious serenity I had heard old-timers share about in meetings. For the most part, I was loving life.

One night, I went to a lecture given by a disciple of a then-fourteen-year-old guru from India who was said to offer true knowledge and awareness of who we really are. His meditation techniques were directed at achieving a personal awakening. As an addict, I always go for anything that sounds like it can produce an instant rush. One of his main disciples, or mahatmas, was in New York on a worldwide trip. So I figured I would fly to New York and get that knowledge. I was willing to go to any lengths. My open-mindedness knew no bounds when I was inspired and driven by the spiritual realm. I checked around for good airfares but decided it would be a lot easier to see him when he was scheduled to be in San Francisco. I would practice patience, and "God in human form," as he was proclaimed to be, would ultimately come to me.

At a morning twelve-step meeting, I announced I was headed for San Francisco. I filled up my gas tank and headed north on Highway 101. In early recovery, decisions are sometimes difficult to make, and even harder to follow through with in action. It seemed like some visions of guidance were followed by a blurred focus, and what had been a chorus of my faith was easily drowned out by that whispering, ever-present fear. I was cruising along in my van, listening to inspiring music, when all of a sudden my head took over. The mental doubts began: *What are you doing? This isn't going to work. What if you can't find these people in San Francisco?*

I listened to those mental doubts for most of the day and used a whole tank of gas going back and forth over a twenty-mile stretch of highway up the coast. *I'm going. No, I can't go.* I kept turning around, heading north and then south. Like my European adventure, I really never got anywhere. I kept watching the movie in my mind, projecting the event over and over, as I literally circled around in my sputtering van.

I went back to a meeting that night and told people about the insane day I had spent on Highway 101. Some laughed, some shook their heads and rolled their eyes in disbelief, but they all understood exactly what I had just needlessly put myself through. It all worked out a few weeks later when this guru's lecture was to be held in Santa Barbara, so a group of us headed the sixty miles north. My sponsor Brandon, Evelyn (the woman whose garage I had rented), and my friend Mike all piled in my van and headed to Santa Barbara for the two-day meditation workshop. We sat in a large auditorium and listened to lectures on this meditation technique, and then the time came to receive the initiation, when they come by and give each person the experience by touching him or her on the forehead, between the eyes.

When the mahatma came by me and touched my third eye area, I experienced a beautiful vision: The young guru's face was in the middle of my third eye, which actually looked like an eye. White light emanated from the middle, with purple colors surrounding it. The vision of the third eye still appears at times in meditation after this initial experience.

I didn't have an instant spiritual awakening, but it seemed like a vast, colorful astral television, in which I rose above my current dimension. Today I know that astral TV experience isn't necessarily significant; what matters is that I show up for my Eleventh Step (Step Eleven is the prayer and meditation step) each day and practice just being mindful of my breath going in and out. When practicing that, I'm present in the moment, and being present is really all there is. It's a beautiful and wonderful experience. Truly being there brings unimaginable joy.

Seeking a spiritual life had become my highest priority, but I was new in recovery and still had a lot of personal growth ahead of me. I think it was good at the time not to know just how much growth would be needed. I was allured by the mystery that seemed to call me. More and more I was beginning to see I was not my paranoid fantasies, and the "what ifs" were unfounded. I was beginning to see I was in fact the *beneficiary of a conspiracy in my favor*! My life was starting to hum and resonate with an old magic that was exciting and new to me. God was all around me, and I felt His presence even more at twelve-step gatherings.

I went to twelve-step meetings and to some *Satsang* meetings of people who followed the young guru. They played music and sang great songs, and we all meditated together. It was awesome. My work in the Twelve Steps and my personal spiritual beliefs had unified into one stream of information. At times in meditation it felt like I was grabbing onto a lightning bolt, the divine charge overwhelming me.

I met a couple, Joe and Sharon, through Laura. Sharon was also a spiritual seeker, and she went to *Satsang*. She was a lovely lady with long hair who wore beautiful, flowing clothes, completely appropriate for the times. Somehow, the energy radiated between us. I was lonely and watching Laura date other men, so I went for it, and Sharon and I began sleeping together. She would come to the construction site where I was working in Brentwood. We ate lunch in my van and then closed the curtains—right there in busy Brentwood—for a bit of afternoon delight.

One night after *Satsang*, I dropped her off down the street from her house and drove to my parking place to sleep by the ocean. After settling in, I heard a car pull up next to my van. All of a sudden, the back door swung open and I saw Joe. He had found out; *they always do*. This was a huge crisis in my early recovery. I had to make amends for my inappropriate behavior. It taught me about honesty, one of the basic requirements for living the spiritual principles of the program. Sleeping with someone else's wife certainly wasn't honest. I was learning another valuable lesson about conscience and doing the right thing for the right reason. Sometimes an awakening of the spirit seems painful at first, and this was surely one those times. The value of a sponsor and network of men in my life I could trust was now apparent, and in cases like this could literally be life-saving. I knew the disease of addiction spoke to me in my own voice; now I had learned it did a frightening impression of God's voice as well!

I began to think about returning to Hawaii. I had talked to Tom, who was living with his wife, Colleen, in Kailua on Oahu. On June 19, 1972, I left for Hawaii, where I turned eight months in recovery on June 20. I was back to where it had all started.

It was wonderful to be back in Hawaii, where my heart and soul have always felt at home since my first trip there in 1962. It was the ground zero of my surrender, and I now viewed it as my sacred home. Within a few days of my return, I decided to head out to the North Shore. It was exciting and strange at the same time. While visiting some friends, I had to call Tom M. because I had this feeling that I should smoke a joint or something. Although I wasn't around drugs, I was re-experiencing my old feelings of living in the area. In early recovery, I was surprised at what could bring on a using thought, and at times it seemed like anything could be a trigger. The monkey that was once on my back had now relocated to my brain, but I knew what to do: call another clean addict. I called Tom and talked about it, and once again I seemed to be okay. Once again, I got through it clean. What a gift of healing the program had given me: willingness to share what is going on inside.

On August 28, Flobird arrived back in Hawaii from her trip around the world to carry her message of hope to addicts. It was wonderful to see her again, especially since I had over ten months in recovery.

This is where my real journey with Flobird began. My first three years of knowing her, I was bouncing in and out of the program. Now I was mindful of being on the spiritual path of recovery, and Flobird was the channel that introduced me to the program. I would say in the twelve-step language that she was my sponsor. Even when I was using drugs I had been drawn to the spiritual path. So I began to develop a guru/disciple type of relationship with Flobird, which I must emphasize is nothing she encouraged and not how she would have described it. I don't think other people in the group related to her in this way. But it worked for me.

These first months with Flobird after her return to Hawaii were certainly helping to shape these ideas of mine. I loved hanging with her. We ended up living at "The Place" in Kailua. It was a sort of community project for young people. Sensitivity groups, sometimes called encounter groups, which were popular in the early seventies, were held there, and some of us in recovery volunteered to talk with the teenagers who came there. I was offered $200 a month to stay there at night in case of any emergency. I had been living with Tom and Colleen in their small two-bedroom apartment when Flobird returned. She had also lived with us, but when I got the overnight gig at The Place, she moved there with me.

Daily, I visited her room after we both awakened and meditated, and I would talk with her about spiritual matters and about my confusion or whatever was surfacing in my life. I had been a vegetarian since 1966, so I loved making her alfalfa sprout sandwiches and other health food delicacies. Flobird ate mostly vegetarian, but certainly didn't claim to be one. She said all food is pure light changing form, and if someone served her meat, she would bless it and eat it. I loved being with her and serving her. I loved walking into meetings with her. We went to meetings in groups. Her hair hung to her waist, and all her followers sported long hair and beards. We were a colorful flock, and soon became known as Flobird and her birds.

One morning, Flobird told me she was informed in her meditation session that we were headed to the Big Island. She and I were to embark on our first adventure together. Most of our travel destinations came directly from the guidance Flobird received in her daily meditations, a practice I was also learning. She called it "following our hearts." At times it was (and still is) confusing, because sometimes it doesn't make sense, and it isn't always easy to carry out. Most of all, we learned to take no thought of or fear for our lives. Instead, we dared to step out into the world, follow our inner guidance, and act as a channel for love and service to others. I was learning that when I practiced faith, what seemed to be a secret, or at times even weirdly esoteric, would reveal itself to me and could eventually become common and routine in my life. With Flobird, our little group had a great teacher, and she taught by example, walking the walk. Our collective lives were mystically altered with every love-filled lesson.

On October 2, 1972, Flobird and I boarded a plane bound for Kona. We were invited to a coffee plantation belonging to friends, located up in the hills overlooking the ocean. When we arrived we discovered a rickety shack unlike any vision we had previously held from the utterance of "coffee plantation," but it was a house and provided a roof over our heads and beautiful countryside. I found it quite comfortable, and during the day I would help pick coffee beans. This type of work was surprisingly enjoyable, and I would find my mind deep in contemplation as I mindfully picked the beans from the leafy branches.

One beautiful morning, when we hadn't even been there a week, I was contentedly looking out at the ocean, listening to Cat Stevens on my cassette player, when Flobird walked out of her room after meditation and said, "God says to leave this place today."

I queried, "Where are we going? Do we have to leave?"

"You can stay if you want," said Flobird. "God told me to pack up and leave."

I had learned to trust her lucid intuition on these matters, and accepted this gentle but direct ultimatum. I gathered my things, and we hitched a ride down the hill. By the end of that day, I was staying in the most beautiful house I had ever been in, directly across the street from the ocean. That's the way it was with Flobird: Listen to the guidance and dare to step into the unknown, but always with the purpose of carrying the message to the one who is still suffering from any type of addiction. At times we would seem to be almost materially "rewarded" when we would try to help others, but regardless of that I was learning that the magical inner peace I would feel was unexplainable, a spiritual balance that was beyond articulation.

Over the next few years, Flobird and her birds traveled continuously throughout the Hawaiian Island chain, mostly back and forth from the Big Island to Oahu. I made a few trips to California to see my kids and regularly stayed in touch with them.

Flobird would continue to come and go in and out of our lives. At times we traveled together, and other times we met up in various parts of the world. But always, our motivation was to stay clean and carry the message. This was written on the tablets of our hearts from the beginning. Flobird always said we were here to be "world servers."

She was showing me that to be of loving service ultimately meant being a servant of God. It was the only work worth doing, and I was discovering that it was the best gig in the galaxy, though the lessons were hard and at times confusing.

Just like the day I got clean, when I headed for the airport with no money and a mushroom candle and sold it for the exact amount I needed for my plane ticket, this is the way I lived during the years I traveled with Flobird. Money for travel, housing, and food always came whenever we needed it. I didn't have a regular job, but worked at whatever came my way. Airline tickets and money just seemed to appear. We sincerely learned to live in the moment, learning that all the necessities would be provided when it was time. Miracles and supernatural forces seemed to spiral around us, and our lives were full of abundance.

Ever since the day Flobird appeared in my life on the North Shore after she was led to the beach house next door, my life had been filled with miracles. I was learning that His will was always in my favor and things always worked out. This was yet another awakening that Flobird had gently led me to.

On previous trips, Flobird and some of the others had stopped in Virginia Beach, Virginia, the home of the famous psychic Edgar Cayce. We had all read many of his books, and I had always wanted to visit his center to seek enlightenment. In April 1974, we headed out to Virginia Beach. I drove across the country with Tom and Colleen and their baby, Scott. I had never been to the East Coast, and the country was beautiful. As we got halfway though Texas, the countryside began to turn green. What a wonderful experience it was to travel through all those states.

When we arrived in Virginia Beach, we found the Edgar Cayce Center and pulled into the parking lot. At that time it was just an old house, but today it is a huge structure. We drove up a road running along the ocean and looked for a place to stay. After a few miles, we saw a hotel with a sign that said, "The Beachcombers." That was the name of our traveling twelve-step group. Wherever we ended up, we always started a meeting and called it "The Beachcombers Spiritual Progress Traveling Group." We held meetings in campgrounds in Hawaii while we were living in tents, in living rooms of houses we rented, and even in caves on the Red Sea. Beachcombers meetings were open to anyone looking for a spiritual way of life within the twelve-step process.

So here was a hotel with that name—we took this as an obvious sign that we should stay, so we rented a room and settled in. In times like these it almost seemed like God responded with a playful whisper. The hotel was directly across the street from the ocean, and there was a long boardwalk. Virginia Beach had a beautiful vibe to it, and I felt immediately at home. Later, when Flobird arrived, we rented a few houses and stayed in Virginia Beach for several months.

On another trip to Virginia with Flobird and some others, we arrived in town with just enough money for one night in a motel. Cruising around, we found a motel called the Aloha. The synchronicity seemed staggering to our Hawaiian spirits. Once again, we were led to a place to stay by the name calling out to us. We stayed there that night, and the next morning we told them we had no more money. The owner said, "If you paint one of the rooms for me, you can stay another night." So Tom and I painted a room every day for the next couple of weeks.

We had free rooms, we made a bit of money, and I had my first experience as a painter, work I ended up doing for years to come. I worked my way around the world, and wherever we went I found painting jobs. Later in life, I ended up owning a painting company with fifty employees and operating on three different Hawaiian islands.

During our first trip to Virginia Beach, we went to a famous psychic named Joy. I had never visited a psychic before. This seemed to go along with our lifestyle, and I was curious about the unseen.

Even Flobird went. Joy was actually a very tuned-in lady who had a lot to say. I got into a psychic addiction for a number of years after that. I seemed to need one to make every decision, which became rather ridiculous. You would think over the years I would have been warned about this future compulsion...by a psychic! I guess it would've been bad for business.

There are two questions everyone wants to know the answers to when they visit a psychic: Where is my soul mate? Will I make money in my life? Relationships and work are the two big questions.

My first reading included a lot of predictions, but one thing the psychic said would affect me for many years to come. She saw me in no more relationships. She said she saw "a marriage to God." When I heard that, tears started pouring down my cheeks. Part of me was elated, thinking that all my past lives as a monk had come to the surface. It just made sense: all the inspirational material I read, my seeking a spiritual path, and being connected to Flobird. I was supposed to be a monk. The other reason the tears were flowing was my thinking, *Oh my God, no girlfriend again—no sex! What am I supposed to do with this?*

With only a few years in recovery, I was vulnerable to all input that came into my life. So I took this information and ran with it. In one sense, I took this prediction seriously, but the other part of me longed for a soul mate. The search for God and the search for a soul mate had begun. I was obviously very confused.

CHAPTER FIVE

SOUL MATES

I know today that the longing for anything is really our hearts longing for union with God. Some call this finding enlightenment, but it took me many years and some painful shortcuts to come to this realization. We want to feel complete, so we look outside of ourselves for something to fill the emptiness. I have always believed in soul mates and have read many books on the subject. The prediction from Joy about my "marriage to God" changed the course of things for a while.

Having an addictive personality, I do nearly everything to the extreme. In the mid-1960s, when I was using, I read a book on yoga that talked negatively about eating meat. I continued to shoot dope, but I never ate meat again. As a vegetarian, I preached about the evils of eating meat—even with a needle hanging out of my arm. In my then-confused understanding and translation of the principle of equanimity, brown rice and heroin were both "natural products."

Consistent with my intense personality, I decided I should be celibate. This wasn't too difficult because I didn't have any girlfriends. I officially took the vow of celibacy and, of course, let everyone know I was doing this, sometimes to the point of annoyance. I stayed celibate for two years and didn't even masturbate. If I had a wet dream, I knew that God got me off.

After my vow of celibacy, I saw the movie "Brother Sun, Sister Moon," the life story of St. Francis, who went barefoot all the time. So I took a vow not to wear shoes, which I kept for nearly a year (I'm surprised I didn't also wear a loincloth). Going barefoot was easy in Hawaii, but not so in the winter months in Virginia Beach. One night, I walked about twenty blocks with snow on the ground, and when I got home my feet were bleeding. I had walked through glass and didn't even know it because my feet were numb from the cold. I had some rather weird ideas of what it meant to live a spiritual life. I had not anticipated the mystical path to be lined with my own bloody footprints.

I had a long beard and even longer hair, and looked like a caveman. So it wasn't surprising I found it easy to be celibate. I mean, did I think some woman would want to date a Cro-Magnon priest? While I was serious about these vows, I also wanted a soul mate in my life. I was torn. My spirit reached for the sacredness, but was I just being a martyr? I finally came to the gradual understanding that rather than "letting go" of the opposite sex, I was in fact clinging to all of them. I now know this is a classic misunderstanding of renunciation or abstinence. I actually went back to Joy so many times that she finally said, "Okay, you're going to meet someone." I might just be the only person who has ever changed a psychic prediction through persistent aggravation.

Whenever Flobird and I arrived in a new place, I immediately checked out the young ladies in the twelve-step meetings. At the end of a meeting, everyone stood in a circle to say a closing prayer. If a woman smiled at me, I went up to her and said, "We have to talk about our relationship." I was so intense and needy that I destroyed any chance of a relationship. My desperation was almost like fragrant incense, and most women would catch this scent and sidestep me altogether. Once, while taking a shower at a friend's house, I noticed a stack of *Playboy* magazines in his bathroom. I knew if I opened one of them my celibacy vow would be over, so I didn't. I managed to stay celibate, with no masturbation, for another day, my dreams that night a little drier.

After about two years of celibacy, I was feeling a bit confused about the commitment I had made. Being truthful within myself, I knew I wanted to be in a relationship, so I counseled with one of my friends in the group, since Flobird was not living with us at the time. We had a heart-to-heart talk, and she suggested I write about it in a Fourth Step format. Steps Four and Five suggest we write out an inventory of character defects, strengths, and weaknesses. After putting it all on paper, we read it to someone. We talked more about this commitment I was now questioning. She told me, "Tom, just go masturbate and move on."

That's what I did, and it gave me the freedom to get honest with myself about wanting a girlfriend. Almost everyone in our traveling group was in a relationship except me. I continued to read books about finding your soul mate, but spent the first eight years of my recovery without a long-term relationship. After letting go of my celibacy vow, I had a few girlfriends here and there; but it never worked out because of the intensity of my personality.

Being single and living like a monk amplified the way I viewed my relationship with Flobird as the most important one in my life. It became more apparent to me that she was my guru. Once again, she would never have said or done anything to approve or disapprove of that title. Since I saw myself as her disciple and found much joy in service to her, being single did seem appropriate.

I went back to wearing shoes and became honest about wanting a woman in my life. The longing for a soul mate remained strong.

I was obsessed with connecting with a woman. My friends said, "Tom, first you have to give up that desire, and then it will come along." Of course, everyone who gave me that advice was in a relationship, so it meant nothing to me.

I remember reading somewhere that it is in the loving that we feel the effects of love; that's the magic of loving, not of being loved. But it was the desire to be loved that was the biggest barrier to my being in a relationship. I didn't have enough self-esteem at the time to believe anyone could love me. Thus, any relationship that came into my life was cut short by my inner obsession to be loved. It seemed like the more I chased what I believed to be love, the further it ran. Jealousy always flared up because of doubts and mistrust that I could be loved, which eventually drove women away from me.

From my own experience, I'm convinced one can be celibate and without a relationship and still find peace of mind and happiness and live a fulfilling life. Although we learn these lessons while being alone, it does not mean we will be emotionally healthy once we get into a relationship. Certain things cannot be worked on until we are in a partnership with the one we love. Whatever we do not resolve in a relationship will keep coming back like an uninvited spirit until it is acknowledged and addressed in the next affair. Conversely, what we work on and correct in our past or present romance may never be a nuisance again. Relationships aren't magic; they are work. It takes walking the path with someone and being able to stick it out to learn the lessons that are essential for living happily with your soul mate.

Most twelve-step programs recommend waiting for a year to establish a solid foundation in recovery before thinking about relationships of a sexual nature. To be blunt, many have learned in the most painful manner that you can't "screw your way" into a new way of living. It's easy to lose yourself in the other person instead of working on your own issues in the early stages of recovery. This is why we have sponsors, people to help us get through the rough spots they have already experienced.

Nothing—and I mean nothing—brings the recovering person to his or her knees faster than a troubled relationship. Over the years, I have experienced this myself and watched many of the people I sponsor go through this. It guarantees surrender faster than anything else. I truly believe that if a person wants to stay in recovery, they will work the program and not use regardless of what happens; but being unprepared for the many facets of a relationship seems to leave people open for the mortal danger of a relapse.

In early recovery, life is mostly about going to as many meetings as possible and hanging out with other people in recovery. But eventually, this is what can happen: The new guy meets the new girl, they hook up, and then the insanity starts. In the beginning, newcomers have no boundaries. The obsession of using a chemical can now shift to the diseased passion for a person.

We are not unique simply because we work a recovery program, and not everyone who winds up in a relationship while in the early stages of this spiritual process is necessarily doomed to failure. Life is a series of relationships—relationships with other people, co-workers, loved ones, a Higher Power, and ultimately, oneself. So in a sense it all returns to honesty, acceptance, and, surely, motivation. What do I want, and am I willing to do the work to get it and ready to accept the consequences of that decision? If so, and if I work closely with my sponsor and seek a connection with God, there may be less of a chance of me harming another or harming myself.

The search for the soul mate is a natural urge. It is only natural to want to be paired up with another. My experiences in early recovery and experiments with "radical celibacy" only brought me more clarity on this truth. It's the desire to love and be loved. Newcomers on a spiritual path, however, tend to immediately cling to the other person in order to fill their longing and sense of emptiness. They have yet to learn that in reality this is a divine longing, not a physical one. The end result is two empty people getting together in a futile attempt to fulfill each other. This has never worked and will never work. It is a spiritual law.

Looking back on my life then and now with the men I sponsor, I have found this to be true. The easiest men to work with are those who are already in successful relationships and have well-paying jobs. In other words, despite having success in their outside world, they still experience profound emptiness. It's easier for them to dive into the spiritual path because they already know that external possessions (people, places, and things) are insufficient. Those not in a successful relationship or with little money, on the other hand, are convinced that if they get those things, the feelings of emptiness will disappear.

I found a book called *The Flowering Tree* by Gladys Jones, a psychic who did unusual readings. She went through a person's entire life, starting at the beginning and using symbols to describe the soul's journey. This book touched my heart. I would underline sections of the book that talked about unrequited love; I would read these sections over and over again, never tiring of my own tears.

I would read things that would describe my tears flowing into a pond, which only the privileged would find deep in the forest. I would read that I was being initiated into a sacred group of people that could be purged of their suffering, that I was being led to a greater love, not known to all men.

The descriptions of an Ancient One said to bide my time, that the acts of my life were not over. I was assured that the finest time would come in the next decades of this life. In those moments, reading statements on love and finding love became a dramatic play of my life, as the visions stimulated more tears.

The longing for a soul mate was so deep within me that I would study similar readings over and over again. Sitting in meditation, I would send love to my other half, knowing that some day we would meet.

After reading that book in 1976, I knew that I had to meet Gladys Jones and have a reading by her. I found out she lived in the L.A. area, and with my traveling between Hawaii and Virginia Beach, I was always going through L.A.

I tracked down her phone number and made an appointment for a reading. I held a Hollywood movie image of what this woman would be like: She would be dressed in a flowing gown and live in a mystical house. The day of my reading, I nervously drove to her house, which turned out to be a rather ordinary place in the suburbs of L.A.

When I met this remarkable woman, she looked like anyone's mother or neighbor. This actually relaxed me somewhat.

My reading from this woman was unlike that of any other psychic I had visited. She walked me through my life, using symbols and characters such as a "sage" or "the mystical one." I could clearly see all the past transitions in my life, including the period in 1971 when I got clean and sober.

She saw a mystical person in my life (Flobird) and a community that I would help start. (It was the year that we were led to New Mexico, and I did indeed start a spiritual community.) As the reading continued on into the years of increased maturity, she saw a peace within about the person I had become and was becoming. She said there was love that would be part of my life, symbolized much like the sacred pool from the book that I had treasured.

Since my long search for a soul mate after getting into recovery, I have found a complete and beautiful love in my life. I have now been with my wife Bea for twenty-five years. She is my soul mate, and our relationship consists of encouraging and supporting each other spiritually. But I had to go through a lot more growth before meeting her, and the journey was worth every step along the way.

CHAPTER SIX

SPIRITUAL GYPSY

The best way to learn any lesson is through on-the-job training, and this is what it was like living and traveling with Flobird. Throughout our travels, Hawaii and Virginia Beach became our homes. I traveled to and from Hawaii half a dozen times a year.

Numerous books about the spiritual life give an intellectual understanding of surrendering and knowing all our needs will be provided for. By surrendering, I mean coming to that place where we quit trying to control everything and everyone around us. Surrender is something I've always reached for on my spiritual path, but just reading and hearing teachings by someone else is not the same as having the experience. Experience means just that—to embrace it, to feel it, to live it. God needs the freedom to move from the mind to the heart.

Living a life of constant travel and learning to listen within for guidance was my apprenticeship program. It allowed me to step out into the universe and trust life, believing each day I would be taken care of. The rent was always paid. There was food every day. Gas money or plane tickets came when needed. The angels seemed to be working in shifts.

We were learning to be spiritual warriors. We watched and experienced miracles firsthand. These years spent with Flobird were to shape my life forever. God knew that our faith was provisional, so He continued providing miracles through Flobird and all of us as we tried to do His work. Lessons became written on my heart, lessons that would be put into action over and over again in the years to come.

Living and traveling in this group situation with Flobird was both beautiful and painful. There were about ten core people who would come and go from Hawaii to Virginia, with many more in both places who would gather around when Flobird was in that area. We all had a common bond of wanting to stay in recovery. We were newcomers on the spiritual path, learning many lessons. We were spokes on the wheel of life, learning to turn in unison.

"Love without a price tag," Flobird told us every day. She talked about practicing unconditional love and being of service to others as the way one finds God. "When serving or thinking of others, we don't have time to think of ourselves," she said. We were learning that this new tenderness we felt when we were of service was indeed a signpost on the path of life that said continue on.

In the early years of recovery, the addict realizes the extent of his or her selfishness and how his or her life is dominated by fear. It was always about "us," and what could we get out of any person or situation. That was the painful part of living with Flobird. This self-centeredness became so obvious to me when I was around her and living in a group situation. I could wake up in the morning and feel so "out of it." Why did I feel this way? I went to bed feeling great, but arose befuddled as to what took place from the time I laid my head on the pillow until rising. I didn't want to see anyone. I felt this darkness hanging over me. The fear would come in waves. It seemed at times that I could be lying in bed and be staring at the ceiling in blissful contemplation, and then turn and roll onto my side and be gripped with the insanity of separation and fear. I would try to trace the footprints of the fear back to its source, but my pain would only intensify. I would be lost in my own mind. Here I was, living in a house with about six other people, but I didn't want to look anyone in the eye. I just wanted everyone to let me be alone. However, the minute Flobird walked into the room, she would speak those famous words, and I just knew they were coming: "What's wrong with you, baby?" She knew everything that was going on with me, and I was forced to go through it no matter what came up. Several responses could erupt from me on days like this. I could just burst into tears, which was probably the best response. Healing begins by letting out those negative emotions. But mostly I would rebel at her and say nothing, or end up swearing and stomping out of the room, although at that point it was too late. She knew the minute she walked in, and then the whole house knew.

There were some days when I could laugh about it. Here we were, a group of recovering people all acting out of our selfish egos, colliding with one another all the time. We couldn't stuff our resentments. I might say some off-the-wall thing to someone, who would then yell back at me or throw a wet dish towel across the room. It was divine surgery taking place without our consent, and we had to experience it in front of everyone. We wanted to be spiritual, peaceful, and full of love, but we were often the complete opposite.

Flobird was like a magnet that pulled this negativity out of everyone. "Uncover, discover, and recover," she said. Flobird constantly talked about getting "out of self and helping others" and "doing something for someone and not getting found out." She knew the rewards of giving love without wanting something in return.

At that time there were few treatment centers, so if an addict wanted our help, we had to bring them home to help them get clean and sober. We couldn't just drop them off somewhere. We lived on the firing line of life in those days. We worked the Twelfth Step out in the trenches. From day one in the program you hear in meetings how important it is to give the message away and help new people coming to their first meetings if we want to stay in recovery, but living with Flobird, it might have been a bit more pronounced.

Everyone in our group smoked cigarettes and drank coffee, except me. So as soon as we came home with someone, coffee was set to brew, and I knew a long night lay ahead. Everyone would get all wired out. We would sit up all night with someone kicking alcohol or other drugs in the house. I'd sit there with my mug of herbal tea, coughing from the smoke with burning, watery eyes, trying to help some smack-addled dude writhing on the couch next to me. It was hard to find my spiritual medicine bag. I really just wanted to open a window, clear out all of the damn smoke, and then make a quick exit. Since I wasn't wired out, I would get really tired and wish the new guy would go to sleep and everyone else would also. Being totally self-centered and wanting to go to bed, I was miserable. But I sat there with nowhere to hide. My bedroom was a sunroom porch directly off the living room and it was surrounded by windows, so there was no way I could even sneak out of the room and disappear into my bedroom. My eyes heavy, the pillows and mattress seemed to tease me from across the room. But I stayed up like all the rest; I showed up and did whatever was necessary to be of service. And guess what? I stayed clean that day and felt better about myself the next morning.

I happen to be a morning person, and I love getting up early and going to bed early. "Why can't someone want to get clean around 6 or 7 a.m.?" I asked. "Then watch me! I could jump into action, with willingness and joy about helping someone!" Never once, though, did that opportunity appear. Either we brought them home, or I would get to bed early and then around midnight or 1 a.m. the phone would ring with a call from someone wanting help to get clean. Not once did

I jump up like a fireman ready to be on call or find myself pulling out of the driveway with tears of joy running down my cheeks; but I did it. I surrendered. I had to. This stuff is life-and-death.

Every spiritual path I have studied emphasizes service, which is essential to living a life of self-forgetting. People in twelve-step programs are so lucky because we have many obvious opportunities on a daily basis to be of service. There are always newcomers at meetings to reach out to. Also, getting to a meeting early and helping set up, staying after and helping clean up, becoming the coffee-maker for the meeting, and many other things within the program offer opportunities besides the obvious one of helping the new person find recovery. We have to learn to get out of self; if not, we use again, and to do that is to die.

During those years with Flobird, we watched her live her life for others, and we felt the unconditional love that poured out of this woman. She taught me that when we speak of being of service, we are really whispering the secret of life. She served with such an uncanny joy and effortless approach that those around her were inspired to roll up their sleeves and learn the art of loving.

Flobird's teachings were always simple. I remember something she once said that affected me deeply. I was in the backseat of a Dodge Dart driven by a guy named Steven. We were driving though Kailua on Oahu, and Flobird was in the front seat.

"Do you know how you can tell when you're making progress on the spiritual path?" she asked. "How do you know you're getting closer to God-consciousness?"

I was excited and asked, "How, Flobird?"

She giggled softly and asked, "When you wake up in the morning, what is your first thought? Usually, it's 'Okay, what do I feel like? What is going on in my life today?' It's 'me this' and 'me that.' You're making spiritual progress when you wake up and your very first thought is 'What can I do for someone else today?' That is being with God. It's that simple, that beautiful. When we get our thoughts off of self, the joy is so incredible."

My personal growth was punctuated with profound teachings by Flobird during our travels. Once, while camping on the North Shore of Oahu, we were all sitting around in a circle. The sun had just set on the horizon. As it disappeared into the ocean, there was a stillness within us all. As the day ended and the sky turned pink, red, and violet, I looked up and the colors reflected off Flobird's tan and wrinkled face. The glow magnified the joy in her eyes. The silence was broken when she asked, "Do you know what God's will is?" Everyone responded with his or her own personal ideas, and some answers sounded rather esoteric.

Flobird smiled and said, "God's will for us is to live, love, laugh, and be happy—and to be a channel for this joy and give it away." This information moved through us like a magical current, with an ancient recognition. This type of spiritual teaching seemed so practical and obvious when we saw it in action through Flobird.

Later, I learned that Flobird's teachings aligned with so many of the spiritual masters, as I was reminded by a story Ram Dass told. Ram Dass had a formal name of Richard Alpert. He was Tim Leary's friend, and they became famous for their early experiments with LSD, but Richard ended up going to India and came back as Ram Dass. He and some other westerners went to India to see a guru. When they finally found him, he was on a hillside talking to a crowd of people. Someone asked Maharaji, meaning Great King, "How do we find enlightenment?" He smiled and said, "Serve people. Feed people." We can't get away from the fact that we have to give love, take no thought for self, and just be a channel of service.

Another example of this same spiritual practice is evident in His Holiness the Dalai Lama's response when asked about his spiritual path: "It is very simple—loving kindness and compassion for others."

During the early 1970s our travels continued. We were in training, learning to live in the moment, and finding out by personal experience that we would be provided for if we just put loving service ahead of all else.

In the midst of our spiritual quests, a member of our group read an article about a place in northern Scotland called Findhorn, a spiritual community on the Bay of Findhorn. Nothing but sagebrush and weeds could grow there, but three people had been guided in their meditation to move there and live in a trailer. Eileen Caddy meditated every morning and started writing down what she received in her meditation, much like Flobird. She was told to plant a garden, which any expert in the field of agriculture would have told her was impossible. But she dared to follow the guidance. Findhorn eventually became world-famous, growing fruits and vegetables larger than anywhere else in the world. Roses bloomed in the snow and cabbages grew to fifty pounds; unbelievable events took place while Findhorn's inhabitants aligned their spirits with nature.

Peter Caddy, one of the founders, came to Hawaii and gave a presentation about Findhorn that we all attended. Because we had already formed a spiritual community, Findhorn ignited the passion within our traveling group. In 1976, one of the married couples in our group left Virginia Beach and traveled west, looking for land to buy. They ended up in New Mexico, about thirty miles into the mountains out of the nearest town, Grants, which is on I-40, seventy miles west of Albuquerque.

The land, which was located at an elevation of 8,000 feet, was a beautiful pine forest that was primitive, with no water and no electricity. They bought a ten-acre plot for sixty-five dollars down and sixty-five dollars a month. A few at a time, we began to join them. At the time I had flown to Hawaii, leaving my van in Virginia Beach, so one of the other couples drove my van to New Mexico, and I flew in later. We had a vision and started our own Findhorn. The progress was gradual, but we were willing and committed and we moved forward.

We had learned through Flobird that the recovery slogan "easy does it" is not an excuse for complacent navel gazing. It still means that you do it!

Our first houses were built quickly, just frames with plywood siding—nothing fancy, but better then a tent. We built a chicken coop, raised chickens for eggs, and used propane for lighting. We hauled water in fifty-gallon drums and installed hand pumps in the kitchen with a hose out the window into the drum. Every time we raised another structure or somehow conquered a seemingly impossible task, we found a new energy and motivation.

Shortly after building the first structure and chicken coops, we discovered we had encroached on neighboring property. This was wilderness country, only about a mile into the forest off the road, but still unmarked wilds. So we bought the next ten acres, which seemed a lot easier than tearing everything down. Then we purchased another ten acres, giving us thirty acres of land in the pine forest. I'm an ocean guy myself (in fact, most in the group were), but the mountains did have their own beauty. Wildflowers in the spring and summer painted the Earth with multitudes of colors splashing across the landscape as far as the eyes could see. The sound of the wind blowing through the pines each afternoon reminded me of the ocean. It was like the Earth doing the OM vibration—OM being the primordial sound of life, resonating throughout meditation practice.

Our only water was in the drums we hauled, so our baths and showers were more like a sponge baths. We found a barbershop in Grants with showers in the back. We were charged one dollar for a shower. It was just like living in the Old West; in fact, I felt like we were pioneers living on the raw land. Sometimes the most basic gratitude is found in the most basic things. In this case, it was the miracle of hot running water and indoor plumbing. We found gifts whenever we looked for them.

That first summer, we built madly, scrambling to raise our houses before that first cold of winter snapped us in two. I had a tent, and my children, now ages nine and seven, lived in my van for the summer. After the kids went home to their mom in Santa Monica, California, at summer's end, it began to get really cold. As a native of Southern California and having lived in Hawaii for the majority of my life, I had never lived in snow country. My house, a twelve-by-sixteen-foot cabin, had a steep A-frame type of roof on it, enabling me to have a loft over half of the downstairs. A ladder went up to the loft, which was surrounded by a railing. A window in the peak of the loft overlooked the landscape dotted with majestic pine trees. I built a bed out of pine logs I found in the forest.

The outside was covered with one-by-twelve-inch, roughly sawed planks. Every Friday I traveled to the lumberyard in Grants to secure necessary supplies to build with over the weekend. I worked as a painter during the week.

I had a wood-burning stove to heat the small cabin, which was a good thing because soon the first snow fell, and the temperature dropped below zero. I remember some winter nights when it plunged to twenty below zero. I'd look up at the ceiling of the home I had built by hand, my breath visible from the frost, and marvel at how life had brought me to this moment. I'd be bundled up in layers, teeth chattering away, but feeling the warmth of joy running through my veins.

I spent months at a time in New Mexico, always bouncing between there, Hawaii, and occasionally Virginia Beach. In the summer months my kids lived with me in the loft, and other times Flobird stayed there.

One of my on-the-job training trips with Flobird took place after we left New Mexico. I had only a little money and a '59 Chevy truck with a camper shell and mattress in the back. It also held my painting equipment, consisting of a couple of five-gallon buckets, a few paintbrushes, and rollers.

Flobird and I left with very little money. We were gone for a little over a month on that trip, leaving New Mexico and ending up in Florida. From there we went to Virginia Beach, then back to New Mexico. Wherever we went, painting jobs would just come to me. This was the mid-seventies, and I ended up making over $800 on that trip, which was a huge abundance to me in those days. We kept showing up and carrying the message of recovery. Flobird said, "Show up, be available, and you will always be provided for."

Those early days on the path with Flobird taught us that in the moment we are taken care of, right here, right now. We would strike a match and the candle would appear. I really believe today that it is okay to have abundance in your life.

One time I drove my truck to California to pick up my children and take them back to New Mexico for the summer. I had enough money for gas to get to California, but not for the return trip. I was sitting on Venice Beach watching my kids play in the surf. All of a sudden my daughter came running to me with a wet wallet in her hand. It had been washing around in the surf and contained sixty dollars in cash but no identification. We had gas money to get back to New Mexico. That's the way it worked. True magic is as real as it gets. Later, after I got a job and earned some money, I gave the money back to Celeste. After all, she was the one who found it; but on that day, she was the channel.

After Flobird left her family and went to Imperial Beach in the San Diego area around 1962, she never had any visible means of support such as Social Security or Medicare. She rarely went to a doctor, choosing instead to try alternative medicine practices. She did see Dr. Whitehouse in Virginia, as we all did; he worked with color healing. He directed different colors of light on our bodies, saying that each different color had its own vibration. He worked with the spiritual body to heal the physical body. He informed us that each body has its own vibration emanating from it; these vibrations, which can be seen by some people, are called the aura. When working with his lights that would correspond with your aura, he would be "sealing your aura." He could detect when an aura had a break or a hole in it. This could be caused by an accident, a serious illness, or substance abuse.

Flobird, who was a longtime smoker, said she could never quit the habit. "It's God's way of keeping me humble and my feet on the ground," she explained. Over the years, along with humility, she developed a chronic bad cough.

In 1978, Flobird and I were in Kailua on Oahu in Hawaii for a while. She decided to travel to the Big Island, but I stayed back to complete some painting jobs. At the time, Flobird was experiencing a great deal of trouble breathing, worse than ever before. Tom M., who was living on our land in New Mexico, said Flobird needed to fly to Texas. Flobird's ex-son-in-law, Pete, who had been married to one of Flobird's daughters, was in Texas at this time at his parents' house. Pete's mother was a registered nurse, and often, during our travels across country, we stopped at their house to spend the night and break up the drive. We thought this would be a good place for Flobird to rest and possibly see a doctor for a checkup.

If any of us were working, we would all pitch in to finance Flobird's trips. It was just our way of giving back. I had just gotten paid when the word was put out that Flobird needed to go to Texas for health reasons. I'm not sure why, but on this occasion I actually rebelled against being asked to contribute. But Tom M. and I eventually agreed to split the price of the ticket and send her to Texas.

When Flobird arrived in Texas, Pete's mom, Shirley, decided she should take her to the doctor. After the initial visit and some tests, the doctor immediately hospitalized her. She had surgery and was diagnosed with lung cancer. But the cancer had spread, so it could not be treated, and they sewed her back up. Flobird was dying. I, like everyone, was stricken with sadness over this news, but I also felt an extreme amount of shame and guilt, since this was the one time I had rebelled about giving up my money. Wow! Flobird was dying and I was caught up in my selfishness.

Some of us headed to Texas. Entering Flobird's hospital room, I broke into tears. The reality hit me that she would be leaving us soon. While in the hospital, Flobird had visitors all the time. People from all over the country flew, drove, and hitchhiked to Texas to see her. She was always sitting in her hospital bed with a huge smile, her hair done in her usual fashion, with the bun on top and hanging long below her shoulders, sending love to all her visitors. They all came seeking final *darshan* with her, one last chance to sit quietly in her loving presence.

The nurses said they had never seen so many people come to see a patient, and many of the nurses found themselves opening their hearts to her and telling her their problems. Flobird's quality of divine love for everyone was entirely natural. It poured out of her, encouraging others to talk honestly and pour their hearts out to her. Flobird's complete lack of judgment of others in all situations enabled her to be completely in the moment with anyone at any time. Her divine love was healing for everyone around her. The nurses were amazed to witness what was happening in Flobird's hospital room, especially upon finding themselves becoming so intimate with this strange lady.

After Flobird recovered from the surgery, she was checked out of the hospital and returned to Pete's parents' house. We all helped out by taking care of her, ensuring someone was with her twenty-four/seven. If she awoke during the night, someone was there to help.

People continued to make the trip to Texas to say good-bye to this woman who had changed their lives so profoundly. She had introduced us to the twelve-step program that saved our lives. We saw how she put love into action and experienced the freedom it produced. We learned to live in joy each moment, no matter what was going on in our lives. Nothing really changed in those last days. She received each visitor with so much joy and compassion, and we were all humbled by this experience. It was amazing to find ourselves totally opening up with our problems. We didn't want to, but our pain just poured out when we were around the 'Bird.

One morning, she awakened and said she needed to get to New Mexico. This was to be her last guidance. On July 14, 1978, Charlie, one of the men who lived on the land with us in New Mexico, and I took off from Texas and drove to New Mexico. Flobird's daughters, Cherie and Marchand, had a bed for Flobird in the back of their car. They headed out at a slower pace with their mom.

After driving all night, Charlie and I arrived in New Mexico in the morning. Tom M. had planned on putting an extra room on his house. He had already installed the pier blocks with his floor joists and put down the plywood. Since we needed somewhere for Flobird to stay, we decided to finish this room for her.

We put our nail bags on and started building. We framed the walls and added some basic siding. Cherie and Marchand arrived a few hours after Charlie and me. For them, the trip was much slower because they had to stop frequently to care for Flobird. They parked their car in front of Tom's house and kept Flobird in the car. We finished the house within a couple of hours after they arrived. We even found a hospital bed; so within hours, Flobird was in a new room with a comfortable bed.

We all took turns sitting with her, and that night she slept off and on, as did the rest of us. At that point, we knew it was just a waiting game. Flobird might live another few months, weeks, or days; we had no idea how long.

The morning of July 16, 1978, I woke up in my cabin and meditated. An overwhelming feeling came over me. I knew I was supposed to leave for Hawaii that day. Celeste, who was almost eleven years old, and Joshua, who was almost nine, were with me at the time because it was summer. The feeling was intensely strong. I told

Charlie about it, and he agreed to drive me to California. He was open to staying or taking me. This was one of the roughest days for me. I struggled with acknowledging this feeling that I had to leave, yet knowing if I did, I would never forgive myself for leaving Flobird. My inner struggle was strong. I had been so close to Flobird the last ten years, had traveled with her (sometimes just the two of us), and she had lived in my cabin with me while she was in New Mexico.

Since I was the only single guy in the group most of that time, it put me in the position of being with Flobird maybe on a different level than the rest of the group members. I had established a very close, personal relationship with her. She was my spiritual teacher/guru and I was her student/disciple. I carried this strongly within me. Regardless of whether it was true, that's how I perceived it. Maybe that's why I was unable to hook up in a relationship with a woman. I thought, "I'm the only single one in the group. I have to care for Flobird."

My inner turmoil on this particular morning was so painful. Was it not what Flobird had taught me all these years? She said to follow my heart, my inner guidance no matter how unconventional it seemed at the time—I should dare to follow it. Yet this guidance was telling me to leave this holy person who had touched my life in a way no one had ever done before. Was I truly supposed to leave this woman with whom I had felt so connected? How could I desert her in her last weeks on the planet? How would I ever live with myself?

As this inner torment went on, I talked to many people about it. Charlie was open to leaving, but the decision was mine. Was I ready to follow this guidance? We were all in Flobird's room that afternoon. She had been sleeping, with labored breathing, and floating in and out of consciousness the entire morning. At that particular moment, she seemed to be sleeping okay. People began quietly leaving the room, until just Flobird and I remained. I sat with her in silence, trying to listen within, trying to find peace in this guidance that said I was to leave the land that day. Quietly I walked out the bedroom door and sat in a chair right outside her room, where there was a window on the wall looking into her room. That window previously looked to the outside, but now it looked into the room we had haphazardly tacked onto the end of the house. I peeked in to check on her, then settled back down in the chair.

I became quiet and went into meditation. While sitting there listening within, a vision of Flobird came to me. I saw her lying in bed with her body surrounded by light. The light was open at the top, resembling a channel or funnel shape at the top of her head.

All of a sudden, I got chicken skin, goose bumps, vibrations—whatever you want to call it—my whole body began to vibrate, all the hairs standing on end. The vibes were so strong I felt almost numb. As I was enveloped in the vision, Flobird began to rise up and out of the channel of light, or her spiritual body did. Her physical body was still lying on the bed, but her spirit body rose upward. She was dressed in white and wore her favorite lipstick, called "Love That Red." She had the biggest smile on her face, and she was glowing.

The vibrations continued to rush through my body. Not knowing what was happening, I jumped up out of the chair and looked in the window. There was a mist in the room. I opened the door, and Flobird was gone. Her physical body remained, but she was gone. She had passed in a glorious way I was privileged to witness. I immediately called everyone, and we all gathered around her bed. We couldn't believe it; our beloved teacher had left her body.

Within the hour, Charlie, my children, and I packed his van and drove away. I couldn't believe I was following the guidance I had that morning. Yes, I was supposed to leave New Mexico and head for Hawaii. I had not deserted Flobird.

Flobird loved rainbows. "After I leave my body, look upon a rainbow and know that it is me," she said. That day in New Mexico was sunny and clear, but as Charlie and I pulled out of the land, we looked back to see the most beautiful rainbow arching over our land. We just looked at each other and left in peace.

About six months after I first met Flobird in 1968 at Sunset Beach, she was guided to go to Maui. Before leaving, she wrote a note in one of the first books she gave me. Part of that note reads like this:

"If I do not go, the holy comforter will not come. Go within your own heart, the Christ of God awaits your call; and when you turn to Him, He always answers. Accept His answers, patient little ones. God loves us and waits for us to accept all His love. I'll be with you always. Think of me, and I'm with you. If you believe in me, you believe in the Father who sent me. I'm in you, you in me, and we in the Father. God is all there really is, pure light manifesting in His colored lights by vibration of His word. Our word does not return to us void. OM, AMEN."

For ten years I was taught many lessons, some of them by example and some by experience. I was on my way to California and then Hawaii, with my two children and just enough money for plane tickets back to the islands. So it was; the adventure continued. The teachings were in my heart, and the seeds were planted. Flobird was now gone, and it was time for me to go live her teachings.

CHAPTER SEVEN

ON WE GO WITH
THE COSMIC SHOW

The first summer after Flobird died was like walking out of my cave in the Himalaya mountains, after years of isolation, moving slowly back into the world. I acknowledged thoughts and desires I had shoved deep down, denying my humanness. I have no regret about that, as I was able to spend time getting clean and traveling with Flobird—experiences most people never have. The seeds she planted within me are still sprouting and growing. I know that everything I did with her was perfect, as it was done in the course of developing a spiritual life. The brilliant light she helped illuminate within me would never fade, but its radiance would surely change shape and direction. The memories are precious to me today: staying celibate for two years, going barefoot for a year, and fasting for up to ten days at a time. Traveling continuously, despite the absence of money, and living in tents, vans, pickup trucks, and mansions on the beach—the richness of those experiences is wonderful. They only deepen and grow in retrospect, as I am repeatedly given the gift of sharing these moments with others on the path.

Being in my first eight years of recovery, it was time to put all of the program's twelve-step teachings into action. I had been blessed to spend those ten years with Flobird and was ready to practice what she had taught me.

After driving to California with Charlie, my kids and I boarded the plane on July 18, 1978, and arrived in Hawaii. We stayed at Steven and Susie's our first night. They were both part of our group that had traveled and spent time in Virginia Beach and New Mexico. I had stayed with them in Hawaii on many other occasions. It worked out well since they had a son, Kevin, who was around Celeste and Joshua's age. But this time, they said I had to find another place to stay. We were able to spend a few nights, but had to find a place to live. That first night back in Hawaii, finding out that we couldn't stay there left me a little fearful. What would I do with two kids, no money, and no place to stay? My daughter Celeste was sick that night, which made me feel even more vulnerable. My first adventure without Flobird seemed like falling through a wormhole into an unfriendly galaxy. I couldn't help feeling that maybe I had made a mistake flying to Hawaii with my children, with no preparation or money. Yet I knew when I awoke that morning I was supposed to leave New Mexico and head for Hawaii; so I did. But this was a very uneasy first night. This would be one of many experiences I would find in the years to come. Following our hearts is not always easy, especially in those times when our mind skips to the next moment and tries to translate a once clear and guiding message. In fact, it can be very difficult at times, but always in hindsight, it is made very clear we are led by the love and care of this universe. Where He guides, He will provide.

At a meeting the next night, everything began to unfold. The way was being cleared for me. I met a lady who was headed overseas for the summer and needed a house sitter. The next day I went to her house to talk with her about it. I found her living in a beautiful three-bedroom house on a hillside in Lanikai, a part of Kailua. As I walked into the living room, my attention was immediately drawn to the panoramic view of a turquoise ocean. One entire side of the house consisted of windows. Gazing out the windows, I could spot the friendly waves of the ocean calling me home. It was only a five-minute walk to the beach. Lanikai Beach has consistently been voted by tourists as one of the most beautiful beaches in the world. So here I was on my first solo adventure, and God blew my mind with His abundance. This was one of the most beautiful houses I had ever been in; totally furnished, including cable TV, which was something of a luxury in 1978, and it was where I was to live for the summer. Whenever I smiled, the universe would smile back.

I called Charlie in California and said, "I have this wonderful house for the whole summer; come on over." Charlie had grown up across the street from Flobird in the earlier days, when she was known as Florence. Charlie had been seeing Flobird's daughter Marchand while they were in high school. He later took off on his own, traveling around the world, but had stayed in touch with Marchand. After returning to the U.S., he got in his van and headed toward Virginia Beach in December of 1975 to visit Marchand, and he walked into our lives. I had felt an instant connection with Charlie from the first moment I met him.

He arrived in Hawaii a few weeks later. We started a small painting business and began making some money. When we weren't working, we were at the beach. If it was cloudy in Kailua, we headed for Waikiki Beach, a popular area where people in recovery would hang out. It was fun to go there and socialize with everyone.

Since the time I had broken my celibacy, I had a few girlfriends but the relationships never really lasted more than a week or month.

Again, I wondered if it was because of my guru/disciple relationship with Flobird, or just karma. Was it the divine plan that I couldn't really be in an intimate relationship while she was alive? I thought so, but who knows?

Now that Flobird was gone, I had a feeling that maybe I could have a girlfriend and make some money in life. I do believe I had stuffed these entirely human and natural feelings. Now my spiritual life was changing, which I later learned is typical for people in recovery. I began to discover that this new adventure included giving myself permission to earn money, to wear clothes and shoes that were not full of holes, and to someday have a wife—that I could be part of the world and still be very much on a spiritual path. Up until this time, I believed that being spiritual meant I had to live in a cave, travel the world with Flobird, and never own anything nice. She didn't teach this to me, but I believe I had possibly been re-experiencing my past life as a monk. Did I really ever live a life as a monk? I can't say, but I certainly had these ideas that seemed to be deeply embedded in my heart. To this day I have visions of myself wandering through India barefoot and seeing where life will take me.

I started dating one of the program women I met on the beach, which was unusual for me. I wasn't in love, but was "in heat," admitting that "Hey, I really do like to make love; this is fun." Of course, along with any relationship come emotions and conflicts that you cannot escape. Once you're in an intimate relationship, feelings and issues arise that you were never aware of before.

Over the summer, I earned and saved money to buy my own car, and actually dated my woman friend for more than a week. It was all a lot of fun.

After the summer, my children returned home to California. The woman who owned the house was still overseas. She had decided to put her house up for sale. In the meantime, Charlie and I still had a home, and we took it one day at a time.

Before coming to Hawaii, Charlie had met a girl in Southern California named Erin, a friend of his then-girlfriend Annette. Erin came to Hawaii to visit and met us one day at the beach in Waikiki. I was still dating my friend at the time. Erin was staying at a hotel in Honolulu and traveling by herself, so we invited her to stay with us. We all hung out together, attended meetings, and went to the beach. Occasionally, I spent the night in town at my girlfriend's house. Charlie and Erin would pick me up in the morning and we would spend the day together. We were three friends living comfortably in the same house. This could have made a great TV sitcom.

Erin was blonde, tan, and loved the sun and beach. I had an attraction to her when we first met. She was born on February 9, and I was born on February 8. Although there was a twelve-year age difference, we were very much alike. We met in September or October of 1978. Things started to change, and I broke it off with the woman I had been dating and became intimately involved with Erin. This quickly led to our marriage on February 10, 1979. So February 8, 9, and 10 were days of celebration in our relationship.

Erin and I stayed together for about six years, which was an important time in my life. For the first time since getting clean, I was in a long-term relationship. A woman stuck it out with me long enough for some of the insanity and insecurity to be worked out. If I could nominate her for being a romantic saint, I would. You can learn certain lessons by living alone, being celibate, and feeling fulfilled by yourself. But there are things that come up in an intimate relationship that will never come up while you're alone. Those six years with Erin gave both of us the opportunity to experience this.

During that time, I learned a powerful lesson on my spiritual path—the danger of complacency, which is subtle and doesn't happen overnight. It slowly creeps in and pretty soon is a part of you. I began to put other things ahead of my spiritual life, which had been based on the twelve-step principles, going to meetings, being of service, and sponsoring other men. After I got married, I stopped traveling as much, began working steadily, and spent time with my wife. These are all good, expected activities when we get into recovery. We are supposed to become productive citizens and healthy people with jobs and successful relationships. Erin and I became long-distance runners, competing in marathons and races of all kinds; this required getting up early and training every day before and after work.

Before long, I was missing meetings because I had to get up early to run. Or I stayed home so we could make love. I gave newcomers my phone number, but told them, "Give me a call, but not too late because I go to bed early to get up and run." I was slowly putting up a wall around myself. This happened so subtly that I had no idea it was happening. I found myself not sponsoring anyone and holding no service positions in my twelve-step program. I still went to several meetings a week, but began to feel separated from others in the program, despite being in recovery for more years than most of them.

Eventually, Erin and I started having problems—she was younger and had her own problems that could have contributed to the emotional pain—and we came to the conclusion that it was time to end our relationship. I found myself with a huge hole in my gut because my wife had become my Higher Power. I had placed my dependence on her and put her before my spiritual path. This was a powerful wake-up call on the fallibility of the human realm, an area that can only be navigated with an even deeper practice of surrender. At that time I had been in the program nearly fourteen years, and I felt like I was brand-new. In hindsight, this was the best thing that ever happened to me because the pain forced me to get back on the path like I never had before. The gift of desperation that had originally brought me into the program had transformed, reappeared, and saved me once again from myself.

Flobird was gone. Erin was gone. I had separated myself from the essence of the program, the Twelve Steps, and I was in terrible emotional pain. There were times when the insanity was overwhelming. I would drive by Erin's new house, look for her car, creep up, and try to look in windows just so I could get a glimpse of her. The obsession had simply changed disguises. What had happened to me? I was back at Step One all over again. I found myself reaching out for help at one of the twelve-step meetings that dealt with family and relationships. At the end of the meeting, after hearing me rant and rave about this emotional pain, a man named Bill came up to me and gave me some literature on the steps. "You need to work the steps again," he said.

Bill became my sponsor. He walked me through the steps again, starting with Step One. It was a fascinating experience, and the most powerful one since coming into the program. During my years with Flobird, she had planted many seeds in my heart. But then she had to leave, and when the time was right those seeds would need to be watered so they could grow. Bill carried the water can that allowed this beautiful garden to begin to grow within my heart.

I was so beaten up emotionally that I was totally teachable, and just found myself showing up and following directions. This was a powerful turning point, and since that time of going through the steps, my life has taken a quantum leap. I now know that the profound personality change that takes place when we first come to the program has to be a continuing effort. Working the steps brings about this most wonderful change, but it must be ongoing. We must surrender to change or we become stagnant; we become complacent. We become robots, simply going through the motions of life. Complacency is a lazy, tired form of fear.

It has been over twenty-four years, and I have been through the steps many times, always reaching for the principles behind each step. I found out that I don't have to be beaten down to work the steps. I can work them when my life is beautiful. I can pick subjects to focus on when working the steps. With each step in the process, I become freer and more awake. It is truly grace.

CHAPTER EIGHT

SHOWING UP

Working through the Twelve Steps with Bill brought me once again to the realization of the profound change that the steps induce in our lives. I was being led in a new direction. What I found out is that I just have to keep showing up. I had gotten to a point of not believing I could help people by saying or doing the right thing, or perhaps I selfishly didn't want them interfering in my life. Looking back, I believe both were true. Both were trapdoors carved out of selfishness and indifference. The concept of just showing up took all the pressure off. That was my deal with God: I just show up for life. I started asking God in my morning meditation to send people to interfere in my life. At one point in my recovery, I was too self-centered to even think those words, but now I could say it and mean it. All I had to do was show up.

This newly found principle gave my life direction and became a turning point during this session of working the steps. Another esoteric mantra had been revealed to me: "Show Up." For the first time in a long while, I was comfortable letting people in. I discovered I had the ability to be okay with someone "interfering." I started to experience a deep joy when working with and thinking of others. It took away the thoughts about me. I started to become a magnet to other people in recovery. They would ask for my guidance and want to work the steps with me. Deep in my heart, I understood my basic responsibility was not to "fix" someone. I didn't have to have all the answers to someone's life. I just had to remain present with them when we were together and share my personal experiences about staying clean in spite of life's ongoing problems. Most of all, I was available to walk with them through the process of the Twelve Steps. On one level, I had simply learned that for every moment I spent helping someone else, it was one less moment spent locked in self-obsession. On another level, there were times I would walk away surprised at how alive and filled with loving energy I felt after helping another. But I must give credit where it is due. It was simply God using me as a willing instrument and vessel. I was in His presence.

I was living alone at the time and loving it. I wasn't seeking a relationship. I slipped back into the monastic groove with the slightest nudge, but this time I didn't have to sleep on a bed of nails. I continued writing out each step because I wanted to continue growing. In the past, if a relationship ended, I desperately sought to casually fall into bed with someone so the emptiness would go away; not this time.

There was a meeting once a week that was held in a friend's house. As I entered one evening, I found my way to a seat. The living room was overflowing as people filed in. Indirect lighting and softly glowing candles brought on a feeling of peace and safety within the crowded room. With the meeting about to start, I looked up as a woman came through the front door. She was tall and slender; her hair was black and pulled to the side as it hung over one shoulder; her olive skin was unmistakably beautiful. She wore black pants and a blue, Asian-patterned blouse. As she moved to find her seat, I found my eyes following her. I felt my heart skip a beat as she brushed past me. I wondered who this exotic woman was.

Not approaching this woman after the meeting was most likely out of shyness more than spiritual resolve. Yet the vision of this woman moving past me that night kept appearing in my mind's eye. Who was she, and would I ever see her again?

I was approaching my Eighth and Ninth Steps, which are focused on making amends. I had a feeling I needed to leave Hawaii for a while, so I talked to Bill, and he agreed it was appropriate for me to leave for the mainland in order to make amends to my soon-to-be-ex-wife, Erin. So I shipped my truck, with my mountain bike in the back, to California and spent six months on the mainland. During this time, I didn't see Erin, but made amends on the phone. I did not try to see her or bother her about our separation. Although I still had feelings for her, amends is changing behavior, so staying detached was probably healing for us both. My ultimate amend was in learning to truly let go, to actualize an even deeper love for her by freeing her from my heart, which had become a captor. I clearly knew I had to be alone for now, and she had made her decision to move on. I surrendered to what is, and peace was my gift.

I ended up driving across the country, spending time in Virginia Beach with old friends, with no pressure to be anywhere at any time, and just letting life happen in the moment. I was a feather in the breeze. Virginia Beach had always been a special place, and I had not visited there in years. I enjoyed daily bike rides on the boardwalk, walking on the beach, and letting the waves of the Atlantic Ocean splash on me as I walked barefoot through the surf. Riding through the woods on the many bike and hiking trails and visiting the Edgar Cayce Center daily filled me with a sense of joy as I browsed through his readings on every subject. I also took time to sit in the center's meditation area, seeking quiet contemplation. I embraced just showing up in the moment. The time came when I knew I had to leave, so I started my trip back to the West Coast, but then decided to go up north for a while. I enjoyed driving around the country, going to meetings. It was a healing time.

Once after attending a meeting in Northern California, a group of people from the meeting went out dancing. We danced for hours, just having fun and enjoying recovery. As everyone was saying good-bye, a woman I had been dancing with asked me to come over to her house. So, I did. Then she asked me to spend the night. So, I did. After all, I was practicing just showing up for life and where it took me. It was a lovely evening, for sure, but I experienced a valuable lesson that night: I could no longer be okay with sleeping with a woman I'm not in love with. She was a beautiful woman and she was the aggressor, and yet just being a physical fulfillment fell short. The spiritual connection was not there, and the emptiness can only be filled by spirit. Something in my heart said, "No." The "friends with benefits" just didn't work for me. That was the first and only time since my marital separation some eight months earlier that this happened. It was one of those almost indescribable times in my recovery when the transformation in my true being was almost alarming, a thunderclap of the new.

The time came when I knew it was right to return to Hawaii, so I left my truck on the mainland with my first wife Laura and our kids. Celeste was now old enough to drive, so I figured she and the family could use it. Besides, I would be returning to visit with them, so I headed back to Hawaii.

I completed my Eighth and Ninth Steps, went to meetings, and continued to work the last three steps with Bill. Right after I returned to Hawaii, an old friend, Eddie, called me and told me that the woman who had taken my breath away at a meeting wanted to go out with me. Her name was Bea. I hung up the phone and called her immediately. I never would have called for that first date if Eddie hadn't prompted me. My head would have said, "She is way too pretty." We had our first date on November 1, 1985. We went to dinner before the Saturday night meeting. We then took a walk on Kailua beach, holding hands as we walked in the moonlight, barefoot in the soft sand, the moon reflecting off the water, guiding us. I found my heart relaxing as Bea's loving essence reached inside me. I felt so comfortable. We talked freely about spiritual matters, finding we had a lot of the same ideas in this area, both leaning toward an eastern philosophy. I saw in that evening that this woman was not only breathtakingly beautiful, but also highly intelligent. As we have reflected back on that first night, we can both say there was love at first sight. It has now been twenty-five years, and we are still together. Of course, we have had a lot of things to work out, but I love her more each day. Any time she walks into the room, she still takes my breath away.

When Bea and I first dated, I was fourteen years into my recovery. She only had ten months. There are no hard-and-fast rules about these things, but it is suggested to wait a year into recovery before making major changes, and messing with newcomers is frowned upon. But I have to say, it seems it was by divine order that we found each other.

So I just kept showing up for life and recovery. At the time, Bea was on welfare, but she soon got a job, went back to school, and eventually entered a doctorate program. She followed the principles we are taught in the program: just show up, sit down, and listen. Eventually she earned a doctorate in psychology and now maintains a private practice in Hilo, Hawaii. She is one the most sought-after therapists for the severely mentally ill. Her talents as a loving healer bless clients with the greatest needs.

Showing up for the moment is what we have both learned to do—and it works. We have been through so many wonderful and challenging times in the last twenty-five years, but going through them in the moment together has always inspired spiritual growth and turned our challenges into new directions and opportunities. When we look back, we can see the challenges have all turned into blessings; it only works by showing up to life each day, each moment, and walking through it all. This simple mantra has been so important: Show up and be present; then grace enters one's life.

CHAPTER NINE

GUIDANCE: FOLLOW YOUR HEART

Flobird said, "One day our actions in life will be more centered on service to others." When receiving guidance, we need to discern things in a spiritual sense to determine if actions are motivated by self-gain or by service to others. If we find our direction isn't self-motivated, then we might dare follow the feeling. One thing I have learned over and over by experience is that when following the heart, the inner movement, it will not always be easy, and at times will be unsettling. It can be like firing a flare into the sky, but then being disappointed when it doesn't turn into a shooting star guiding our every movement. If we keep going forward and completing each assigned task, the purpose is generally revealed in hindsight. The path we take will always be illuminated, even if it is only footlights in front of us, guiding us safely. It takes tremendous courage to move forward without knowing the outcome. We can experience doubt, loneliness, and fear, but always on the other side is a great joy and peace born out of the experience. We must always remember when putting guidance into action, our motive is to serve. This inner whisper will not make sense at times, but other times the sense of clarity is astounding. One key practice is learning to filter out the static noise of our ego until we only hear the still and centering melody of God's will. Living life by following guidance received from meditation is simply a life full of joy, even from the beginning. My life has been a glorious adventure of stepping out into the unknown. By walking forward, with little concern for what others might think of my path, I have developed a deep trust in the process of what is. All shadows will eventually turn back into light.

Carrying the message by listening within came to a halt after I had gotten together with Erin. Erin and I did spend some time in California for a few months at a time, but our travels certainly weren't driven by sitting and listening to the still, small voice. I had gone from being a seeker to being a sightseer. Traveling with Flobird was like being a gypsy; now I was becoming a tourist. In the nine months I spent alone after separating from Erin, my spiritual wanderlust returned. Thus the six months I spent traveling on the mainland and finishing the steps with Bill released my spirit once again. Each morning upon awakening, I would look in the mirror, and there they were: My wings were sprouting. I was a bird again. Birds fly.

In September of 1986, Bea and I had not even been together for a year when I found myself being pulled to London. There was a huge twelve-step convention being held, and I felt I should attend it. My new sense of freedom commanded that I go by myself. In alignment with the way I used to travel, I set off with no prior arrangements for a hotel room or lodging. I pictured myself landing in London and showing up at the hotel on a beam of light, with everything laid out before me. In actuality, I found myself wandering aimlessly with no place to stay, knowing no one, and lost in space.

The first day of the convention started with open sharing at the podium. I was sitting in my chair, shaking. I told myself I was cold from being in London in September, since I was acclimated to Hawaii's balmy warmth. Yes, I was cold, but I was also scared out of my mind. One thing I had learned throughout my years of recovery was to share my feelings, so I felt compelled to rise and, with knees knocking, made my way to the podium to speak. I talked about my fear and my feelings of not fitting in. I admitted I was missing my girlfriend already. Once I did this, the magic happened, and I felt better. More than one addict in the room seemed to nod their head or even chuckle in understanding and agreement. Not only did I feel immediate relief, but many people approached me to thank me. They were feeling the same thing. Once again I knew this program really worked.

My friend Don from Hawaii eventually showed up, and we found a bed-and-breakfast inn (B&B) not far from the convention hotel. I felt a little more secure after a trusted brother and part of my network had arrived. I was hoping that at the very least we could be confused and lost together. I enjoyed the rest of the weekend and met a lot of people. Before leaving Hawaii, we had planned to go to northern Scotland to visit Findhorn, the spiritual community I had heard about in the early 1970s. We had befriended a girl at the convention named Denise, and she joined us on the adventure.

After the convention we drove to the Bay of Findhorn in northern Scotland. The drive north was breathtaking, with meadows stretching across the landscape colored by the many shades of green. Driving through the small villages, with cobblestone streets and old buildings of stone resembling small castles, provided enough visual stimulation to entice anyone to spend a month. We stayed at B&Bs that were the quaintest houses. I was sure they were made of gingerbread, with gardens of colorful flowers and trimmed hedges aligned in perfect symmetry. With every turn of my head, there was another beautiful landscape. It felt like I had fallen into a fable or a wormhole of childhood stories. Was I in the Garden of Eden?

But I was missing Bea very much the whole trip. My longing was so pronounced that I began stopping at every phone booth to call her. At one point she said, "I can't even remember what you look like," indicating she was going through her own difficulties, feeling abandoned and such. Her voice sounded impossibly small over the long-distance connection, which made me want to go back and be at her side. Yet I felt I had to be a bird and go on by myself.

At Findhorn we participated in a program called experience week. The week is designed for visitors to live and work in the community while participating in workshops for part of the day. The rest of the day is spent in service within the community. You could be assigned to work in the garden area, or in the kitchen to help prepare the beautiful and delicious vegetarian meals. We would also help clean the facility. Experience week gave us an introductory course in what it was like to live at Findhorn. After that week Don and I bid good-bye to Denise, who had decided to extend her Findhorn visit. We caught an overnight train to London. From London, Don flew back to Hawaii, but I continued on to Israel.

I knew people in Israel who were in the program and had lived in Hawaii. We spent about ten days traveling around the country, sleeping on the beach of the Dead Sea and the Sea of Galilee, lying on the desert floor while gazing into the night sky as the stars seemed to dance in a spectacular light show. I was transported on a journey into the past. My thoughts and visions swirled in a salty mist. I couldn't help but think Jesus walked on this ground. Jesus had been one of Flobird's teachers. In the beginning, she couldn't even say his name because of old ideas developed from years of attending church and hearing that she would go to hell for saying Jesus' precious name. So she called him Little Boss. She carried a huge oil painting of him and hung it on the walls of each house we lived in. As I lay there in the silence, the gratitude welled up, knowing that Flobird had lived the teachings of this carpenter, and she had, in turn, touched our lives.

In Israel, you will find a church built atop most holy and sacred spots. One such church in Bethlehem is considered the birthplace of Jesus. Walking in, I descended the stairs to the basement and found a star encased in a plaque in the ground, representing the exact spot Jesus had been born. Finding the light muted in the lower part of the church, I knelt in front of the marked area. I sat within the silence, being mindful of where I was, and a feeling of tremendous peace arose within me. As it flooded my entire being, tears rolled out of my eyes. The energy was beautiful. I sat there completely caught up in the experience. Then the transmission occurred; all of a sudden I heard what I thought were angels beginning to sing "Silent Night." Tears continued streaming down my cheeks. Then I seemed to come back into my body and found that a group of people had entered the basement area and had begun to sing. There was no miracle of angels, but it was something I will never forget.

Attending a twelve-step meeting in Tel Aviv was also an experience in itself. The meeting was held in a bomb shelter beneath the busy streets. As I walked in and sat down, I noticed the common literature that hangs on walls in meetings around the world, with only one difference: It was all in Hebrew. I sat next to my American friend, and she translated for me as people began to share. What I find to be so enlightening is that no matter what language people share in, the emotions behind the words are universal. There is only the energy of love, endlessly changing its form. We all talk about the feelings of isolation, despair, and loneliness we felt before finding hope in recovery. My mind moved out of the way and my heart understood completely.

After I returned from my travels in England and Israel, my relationship with Bea continued to grow and blossom. Around April of 1987, we really made the commitment to be together and got our own place in Lanikai, a beautiful beach community in Kailua on Oahu. I had just been asked to speak at a twelve-step convention in Australia. The day of my departure happened to fall on the day we were moving into our new home. I was to be gone for three weeks on this trip. Finding myself once again headed out on my own, I embraced my birdlike spirit. Did I miss Bea? Absolutely! But sometimes the journey in recovery is a solitary one.

I returned to Australia again in September of 1987 for another twelve-step convention, once again alone. Bea was very loving about all my traveling. The point of traveling solo was never to just go somewhere by myself. If I was asked to speak somewhere, I would go. In the program it is very important to carry the message to the person who still suffers. I had learned my job was to show up; God was already there, waiting patiently. So, I went, but I always missed Bea. She never said, "You can't go," but she did get sick of hearing how much I missed her. To this day we laugh about that. Her response is always "I don't want to hear how much you miss me while you're in these exotic places by yourself." Over the years we have both come to the understanding that if I do travel by myself, I try to make it a week or less.

Early one morning in September of 1989, I was sitting in our meditation room, practicing the Eleventh Step. Candles were burning, with the light reflecting off the many crystals placed around the room. A thin trail of smoke floated upward from the incense burner. I became mindful of my breath going in and going out. I focused on my mantra. Thoughts came and went. I didn't hang onto or pay attention to them, but just let them float through my mind's eye. A stronger and more focused thought found its way through the maze of the dancing neurons and appeared on the scene—it was a thought of India. I didn't attach myself to it, but it seemed to stay in the forefront. Then it happened, like it had happened on other occasions. There was a voice within—it came with a vibration that stands the hair straight up on my arms and the back of my neck. What some might mistake as their skin crawling, I recognized as the spirit in motion. I knew in that moment I was being guided to India. Then, like a neon light, the word "Calcutta" appeared. I went out of the meditation room to tell Bea, "I'm supposed to go to India." Her loving response was "Okay, Tom." No matter what she felt about any of this, she has always been supportive.

The guidance was crystal-clear. It said, "Go to Calcutta (now known as Kolkata)." I wasn't sure what the connection was and why I was supposed to go to Kolkata, but I did know that Yogananda had grown up there and that the Mother Teresa Center was also located there. I knew I would love to meet her and be in the presence of a holy woman. I also knew my primary purpose was to find the addicts in India and see if I could find some meetings. However, I had just read an article in a twelve-step publication about some members who had recently traveled to India and found that there were no meetings in Kolkata. Yet my meditative guidance left no doubt that this was to be my destination. The message was clear as love.

The preparations for my trip began. By this time I had about ten employees working for me in my paint company, and for once I actually had money for the trip. I was always taught to go with the heart and trust that all would work out. I was in India close to a month, and the gift was that in that month, my company made more money than I had ever made in a mere thirty-day time period. Flobird's edict of carrying the message and all else will be taken care of proved itself true.

Kolkata is one of the largest and poorest cities in India. When the plane touched down, no tourists got off. I was one of the few westerners with Kolkata as my final destination. After going through customs and walking out of the dimly lit terminal into heat and bright sunshine, it was like being catapulted into another dimension. My senses were attacked with smells and visuals that took a minute to assimilate. Hundreds of people were shouting, holding up signs for taxis, or wanting to carry my baggage. Women with babies in their arms approached me with palms up, begging for money. Finding a cab proved to be quite easy, since there were hundreds lining the street for hire. The black-and-yellow Ambassadors, Ambys for short, crowded the streets. There are approximately 60,000 Ambys taxis, made by the Hindustan Motor Company, in Kolkata, adding to the pollution of the city.

Having done research before leaving on the trip, I knew Sudder Street was a part of town where I could find a cheap room. As I gazed out the taxi window, I was overwhelmed by the poverty I was seeing. Cardboard houses erupted from sidewalks. People were using the fire hydrants to bathe in and brush their teeth. I had no trouble finding a room for $1.50 a night. The room was small and needed a paint job. Being a painter, I noticed that probably nothing in this city had been painted in the last fifty to one hundred years. The bed had clean sheets and the floors had been swept. The bathroom even had a sit-down western toilet—this was a real luxury, as most toilets in India were holes in the floor you squat over. Everything was old but clean. After unpacking all my stuff, I sat there for a minute. I felt lonely and scared, but I remembered just the day before when Bea had dropped me off at the airport. I walked into a restroom after checking in, looked in the mirror, took a deep breath, and said to myself, "Okay, here we go." Was I up for the adventure? Yes.

I wanted to meet Mother Teresa, so I walked out on the street and found a cab to take me to her center. I was dropped off by an entrance to a narrow alleyway. Just a small walk up the street, I found a door. It had a simple sign above it that read either "Mother In" or "Mother Out." On this first visit, it read "Mother Out." I entered the small door and found myself in an open courtyard surrounded by several nuns in white-with-blue-trim saris. The saris were the habits of the Missionaries of Charity, an organization Mother Teresa had started after her calling in 1946. While traveling by train to Darjeeling, Mother had a vision of Jesus. He said, "I want you to serve Me among the poorest of the poor." This inspiration, of course, changed her life forever. In 1948, Mother applied to Rome for the privilege of exclaustration—living outside the convent. This request was granted, and a new order of nuns took the complete vows of poverty and began working with the poor of Kolkata.

I approached one of the nuns walking through the courtyard. I told her I was from the U.S. and would very much like to meet Mother Teresa, if even only for a minute. I explained that just to be in her presence would be such a blessing. The nun smiled at me, with eyes so full of love and compassion that warmed my being with comfort. My loneliness drifted out of me like a warm wind was blowing it away.

This loving sister took me by the hand and told me, as the sign had indicated, that Mother was out of the center at the moment. She asked me if I would like a tour. I exchanged my disappointment for acceptance of the situation. I readily agreed, and we walked up a narrow flight of stairs, entering a large room with folding chairs lined up and facing an altar at the front. It was nothing fancy, but I was astounded to actually be in the chapel at the Mother Teresa Center. I was told there was a service every morning beginning at 6 a.m.

I also mentioned to the sister that I was primarily in India to work with addicts, and was in search of twelve-step meetings. She looked at me, smiled, and took me next door to the orphanage. The building was several stories high. Children are picked up off the streets and find shelter there. They are fed and can attend school within the walls of this safe place. Their faces were aglow, and most sported big smiles with white teeth. They gathered around me and giggled. As I knelt down to say aloha to them all, their joy was infectious. Next we went out to the street and hailed a rickshaw, which is a popular method of transportation in Kolkata. This is one of the only places left in the world where the carts are still pulled by a man, and this is how I traveled from then on. Our next stop was the House of Dying. The sisters go daily out on the streets and bring back many of the dying who live in the open. They give them love and dignity in their last days on Earth. Walking into this large room with beds lining each side, I was reminded of the military barracks from my days in the Navy. Only this place was not a station of regimented precision, but a refuge of impermanence and beauty. As I walked down the center aisle, tears began to roll down my cheeks. Sadness and joy both filled my heart. You could not help but feel the joy, since vast love permeated the room. This love entered every pore in my body and transformed the sadness into compassion. In this moment, true charity took on the deepest meaning for me. I never forgot this experience, and within a year or two after returning home, I would be compelled to take hospice training.

We left there, and I kept saying, "I have to find the addicts." Once again, my lovely guide just smiled at me. Flagging down another rickshaw, we weaved our way through the busy streets of Kolkata with horns blasting and people darting out of the way of cars, motorbikes, and rickshaws. I wondered how it could all possibly work on the busy roads, but somehow it did. The sister took me to a two-story house. It was now about 5 p.m. I had been in Kolkata since about 1 p.m. As we walked up a shaky set of stairs and entered the house, I felt at home immediately when I entered and noticed chairs set in a circle—a familiar pattern of a meeting. I was introduced to a lady named Joann. It happened that her husband ran a rehab center for addicts and alcoholics. Joann was a friend of Mother Teresa and the nuns. My guide knew Joann's husband ran a rehab center on the outskirts of Kolkata, so here I was. The miracle did not elude me, since in one hour a meeting was scheduled to begin right across the street. I was struck with awe. I was led right to a meeting in one of the largest, most crowded cities in the world. My smile permeated the streets of Kolkata.

Walking across the street at the time of the meeting, I still found myself amazed that I was about to walk into a twelve-step meeting. This had to be a divine situation. My own best thinking, planning, or research could not have made this any smoother. As I entered the meeting, which was held in one of the city's schools, I found small desks lined up around the room with about fifteen men sitting and talking. Smoke filled the room and there were laughter and smiles on the faces of these Indian men. One other western man attended the meeting that night. His name was Father Dan Egan, also known as the "Junkie Priest." There is a book entitled *Junkie Priest* about his life. Father Egan worked on the streets of New York City with drug dealers, prostitutes, and junkies. This was his calling to serve God. He was in Kolkata now to meet with Mother Teresa's organization to help the addicts on the streets.

The meeting was probably one of the best I had ever attended. Just the willingness of these men to stay clean impressed me deeply (at that time, there were no women in the recovery meetings, though today there are many women who attend these twelve-step meetings). They could not afford literature. They had just one book with limited information. From that night on, throughout my ten days spent in Kolkata, I was busy going to meetings and spending time with some of the men in the program. They were eager to share about this new life we had all found, of being in recovery and working the Twelve Steps. They had so many questions and so much excitement. Each one just wanted not to use again.

One of the members from the meeting, Seth, invited me to his house. We walked down a lane so narrow I was almost able to reach out and touch the walls on each side. As we came to a door and entered, I found myself in a dark room with light slipping in between the cracks of the wooden walls. As my eyes began to adjust, I saw that the room was about eight-by-ten feet. Benches lined the walls, and the floor was of dirt. This was where Seth and his family lived. I felt so honored and blessed that Seth would bring me to his home. You have to understand, this simple shelter was something to be grateful for with thousands living on the streets. I met his baby and his wife. She was pregnant for the second time, but was strung out on heroin and couldn't get clean. Seth had only eight months clean himself. Going to his house is something I will never forget. When I returned home, it took me several months, if not years, to be able to describe this experience without crying.

One evening Father Egan invited me to join him and some other priests who were meeting to discuss what the Mother Teresa Center could do to help the addicts on the streets. He gave me the address and directions to where they were meeting. I hired a cab that evening to find the meeting place. We were winding in and out of small alleyways through the darkened streets of Kolkata. When driving at night, it is considered rude to have your lights on because of the glare in the eyes of the oncoming driver. That makes sense, but how do they see where they are going? This just added to my trepidation as we weaved our way through the dark alleys. Once I arrived, I felt as if I had been led to a secret hiding place. I sat down with four priests in a round-table discussion. It was such a privilege to be attending something that could be a turning point in the lives of the addicts of Kolkata. My role was to remember throughout discussions that twelve-step programs cannot align themselves with any outside organizations. This is one of the tenets of our suggested traditions. Further, we accept no outside contributions. Thus, working with the priests of the Mother Teresa Center as a representative of twelve-step programs proved to be as big a responsibility as it was an honor. When I got back to the U.S., I had a huge supply of literature sent to India, to the Mother Teresa Center's address, so the twelve-step groups might be assured they would receive it.

They call Kolkata "The City of Joy." I knew why after being there. Even amidst extreme poverty and addiction, I was never fearful. Walking the streets at night to and from meetings alone, with the depression of so much need abounding, left me amazed at the love and joy pouring from every smiling face. When I got home from India, I told people, "You know, I never saw the sky in India." This was simply because there was so much going on all the time right in front of me; I just never thought of looking up.

The day before I was to leave Kolkata and fly to Nepal, I was invited to the treatment center that Joann's husband directed. Seth and a few other men came by my hotel in the morning, and we started our trip to the outskirts of town. I was asked to give a talk for the men in residence. I did so with great enthusiasm, sharing about my life, how I had drunk and used drugs, my experience finding the twelve-step programs, finding a sponsor, working the steps, and finding ways to get into service. My talk focused on the basics of the program and how we don't use, one day at a time. After talking and answering questions—there were always so many questions by these excited and willing men—we were invited to stay and have a meal. I knew before coming to India how important it was to eat cooked food and drink bottled water. I always carried bottled water with me. However, this was a very hot day, and I had finished my water. During the meal of cooked food, I became quite thirsty. They assured me they had a system that filtered water, so being hot and dry of mouth, I drank a glass of water. Oh my, what a mistake that turned out to be!

When I got back to the heart of the city, my friends dropped me off at the hotel. They were to pick me up the next afternoon and take me to the airport to fly out. We all hugged. It had been a good day of recovery. Waiting for me at the hotel was an exciting message from Joann: "Tom, please meet me in the morning at the Mother Teresa Center at 9 a.m. I have arranged for you to have an audience with Mother Teresa. Please don't be late. She has meetings all day." Electricity ran through my body. I was filled with joy at the thought of being in her presence, even for a minute.

Upon awakening the next morning, my eyes opened to a darkened room; I knew it was early. It was the quiet period of Kolkata, even before the Muslims started their morning prayers over the loudspeakers, sending their chants over the sleeping city at 4 a.m. The first thing I noticed in the stillness of this morning was that I felt as though I was getting sick with the flu. My joints were aching, and I felt hot. I got out of bed and headed to the toilet. There seemed to be more immediacy than usual. Within the hour, I knew I was really getting sick. Everything started pouring out of both ends. After a few hours, I became weakened. Only one thing weighed on my mind—I had to somehow get to the Mother Teresa Center. My movements were extremely slowed, and the trips to the toilet continued and were becoming more frequent. I found my way to the streets of the crowded city that was now awake and streaming with life everywhere I looked. I was late getting to the Mother Teresa Center. Mother Teresa was already in her meetings, and by the time she was due to be out, I would have to be at the airport. I was terribly disappointed with not being able to be in her presence, knowing I might even have a spontaneous healing. I was getting delirious by this time. One of the nuns was gracious enough to bring me a signed note from her. I placed it in my pocket and began the journey back to my room.

Upon arriving back at the hotel, I was able to gather my things, and two members from the program came by to help me get to the airport. I could feel I was starting to run a high fever. Seth and my other friend knew what had happened to me. I had drunk the water at lunch the day before, and even though it was filtered, it obviously didn't work for me.

On the way to the airport and while waiting for the plane, the three of us were talking about recovery and how to stay clean. I felt so powerless at times. My new friends had so much to overcome. They had no program literature. They had no books. These things would cost a month's pay in India. But despite all these challenges, here we had people staying clean. They wanted to work. They wanted to support their families. When they got out of rehab or jail, what were they were supposed to do? The full responsibility of a clean and sober life rested on their shoulders. There is no welfare system in India like in the U.S. What was I supposed to say to these wonderful human beings who so much wanted a better way of life? They had nothing in the way of support compared to the standards of recovering people in the U.S.

I found myself saying to them what I would say to other addicts trying to stay clean anywhere in the world. My heart felt heavy; I wanted to give more, but I continued on. "Work the steps. If you can't find a job, get in service each day. If you have some clean time, go to the rehab center daily and talk with the newcomers. Get to a meeting daily. Get there early and set up the chairs. Do these things—the same things required of any of us," I said to them. "Stay clean and life will unfold."

When they dropped me at the airport, I knew this experience had changed and helped me in more ways than I could ever believe. I was also sicker than I had ever been. I slowly found my way to the men's room in the airport, which did not have western-type sit-down toilets, only a hole you squat over. So there I was on my hands and knees, bent over a hole in the floor with someone else's feces still in the toilet, puking my guts out. I tried to summon some faith and humility between the violent spasms of retching, but my spirit seemed more concerned with staying conscious, alive, and upright.

Somehow I got out of the toilet area and to the gate to board the plane to Nepal. After takeoff, I spent the rest of the flight in the bathroom of the plane, which was way cleaner than my previous adventure at the airport. I couldn't even return to my seat for the landing. After we landed, the flight attendants had to come aboard the plane with a wheelchair to help me off. Some westerners assisted me through customs, which I have no memory of, and they checked me into a nice hotel right next to the airport. It was $100 a night, which wasn't in my travel budget, but it was what I needed—modern and clean accommodations. A doctor was even sent to my room once I checked in. There was also phone service, and within a few days I was able to call and connect with Bea and let her know what was happening.

The next day or two were touch-and-go. My fever was still running high. One time I came to and was on the bathroom floor with my head in the lap of a beautiful Indian woman. I had passed out there for who knows how long, and she found me. She was holding me, applying a cold washcloth to my head, stroking my temple with her gentle fingers. Later I learned this lady was one of the housekeepers.

That night or day, I don't know which it was, I experienced what I would call leaving the physical body. I knew what was meant by "the breath of life." We hang on, one breath at a time. I could actually feel the thin thread between this life and the afterlife. I could almost feel I was about to take my last breath, but I knew it wasn't time to do so. I hung on. Past lives flashed before me. I was given messages from God to give to certain people. I believe I left my body for a while. Was it just a high fever and hallucinations, or was it real? I don't know, and I don't care. I just know it was a breakthrough. When I woke the next morning, I was back in my body. The fever had broken. I was so glad to be back. I could still remember the visions and messages I was given. The messages were for five different people. They came in almost a poetic and symbolic form. One was for a friend, a pro tennis player, who was in the program. One of the things I was supposed to tell him was to be of love and service. It occurred to me that those two phrases are also tennis language.

The people from the plane who had brought me to the hotel came by to see me, and I told them I was supposed to meet two friends in Katmandu. Linda and Patti were friends of Bea's and mine who were in the program, and both were nurses back in Hawaii. They had given me the name of a vegetarian restaurant in Katmandu run by some people who also had a small guest house where we had planned to stay. I gave the couple from the plane this information, and they located Linda and Patti, who had been going to the airport daily looking for me, not knowing I was almost dying in a hotel right next to the airport.

I was much too weak to move yet, so it was a couple of days before I could travel at all. I was finally able to leave the hotel with

Linda and Patti and continue my adventure with them, although I was still weak and living on tomato soup. But I was healing—I had made it.

I believe the trip to India was God's will for me. Although it wasn't an easy trip, I grew so much. I gained more faith and trust from the experiences I had on that trip. In hindsight, we can always look back and see the gifts. The guidance was right on.

I was glad to come home after that first trip, but India had an effect on me that has kept me going back. I'm always excited to return, but also always ready to come home. I have been blessed to have traveled all over India. I have taken trains all around, getting off in different cities and working with addicts. I have held workshops on the steps, and I have spoken at several conventions. The twelve-step programs have grown so much there. Recovery has spread everywhere. What a gift to see this happen! Throughout my years of travel to India I have never seen Seth again, but I have heard reports about him. He had gotten a job and was working in the rehab field. The last I heard, he had over fourteen years clean. This is the joy of working with others.

When traveling through India, you can witness poverty at a level most people may not be used to. It has such an effect on your heart. It saturates your being—the side of a postcard one never wants to see. I learned from the writings of Mother Teresa that it is better not to give money to the beggars if all you're going to do is give them the money, meaning they need love and recognition more than the money. So, anytime I was walking on the streets of India in any city, I would be sure I had easy access to loose money in my pockets. I loved walking the streets and sitting down with the poor, who were asking with their hands out. I would stop and talk with them. I would say, "Namaste," which means "The God, the joy, the light in me, salutes and honors it in you." Namaste is one of my favorite words in the world.

I would follow Mother Teresa's thoughts on the poor and acknowledge their presence. I would touch them and embrace them.

Even the lepers, I would hold. Then, only after making human contact, I would hand them money. The smiles of love and appreciation I can still see in my mind's eye. I would always adopt a certain few people if I was in one place for a few days. They would recognize me walking down a crowded street and approach me with such love and gratitude. It was such a gift to be in their presence. The gratitude they had for life was contagious. I had so much to learn from these experiences.

On Bea's first trip to India, we were in Kolkata, so we got a ride to the Mother Teresa Center. As we approached the door, we noticed the magic words "Mother In" on the sign that hung at the entrance. We walked in with great anticipation. As we entered the open court area, there was a small nun talking to another sister. Directly in front of us was Mother Teresa, with no crowds around and no security. She was simply standing there in front of us. This intimate moment of being in the presence of a living saint could have happened nowhere but here in India. She would have been guarded heavily in the U.S., with huge lines to even get a glimpse. I found myself at 6 a.m. mass every morning while visiting Kolkata. Mother would be there every morning, sitting humbly in the back of the church. After the service was over, I would take my turn to approach her and be blessed. Then I would walk home through the crowded streets as families were just waking up, washing in the fire hydrants and getting ready for their busy day on the streets.

I also made contact with Yogananda's family on my trips to Kolkata. I knew from reading his *Autobiography of a Yogi* that he had grown up here, and the house was still in the family. In his autobiography, he described his meditation room called the attic, where he saw his first visions. From there he climbed out the window and ran away to the Himalaya mountains on his search for God. I sat in this room in silence and could feel his love.

One of my favorite moments of guidance occurred when my wife and I were leaving for India in the mid-1990s. We made our reservations to go, but we didn't pay for the ticket until right before leaving. Yet our seats were held for us.

About eight or nine days before we were supposed to go, my business was in debt, so there was doubt about whether this was the right thing to do. I went into the meditation room and closed the door. I sat in silence, asking for a clear message as to whether we were going to India or not. The money situation was not good, but I knew I was willing to go and carry the message. There was a convention in Kolkata, and they wanted me to come speak. Knowing my motive was in the right direction, always coming back to service, I sat there in silence and nothing was coming through. After a bit of time, I blew out the candles and walked out of the meditation room. As I walked out and closed the door, the phone rang. I answered it. It was someone from the Wood Valley Buddhist Temple, which is about an hour from our house. Eight months prior, they had held a fundraiser and we had donated $100. They had just held the drawing, and we had just won first prize—a round-trip ticket to India. There was our answer. We were going to India.

What I have experienced by living with and around Flobird for ten years, plus my own life over the past thirty years since she left, is that these occurrences are common, and actually the way we should live our lives. We must slow down each day and listen. The guidance will come to each of us. We don't have to be psychics, although I guess we are when we let it surface. I am convinced that life can be lived from this place within, where we come in touch with the higher self and can be guided to always be at the right place at the right time.

For me it is so important to remember why I practice meditation. Why do I seek God or enlightenment? Is it for me or is it for the sake of others? I must remember always that I'm here to be of service. We meditate to become clear channels for the love that binds the universe together. Since my first meeting with Flobird, this is the message that has been given to me. Love, in action, is the magic way. All the mystics, gurus, saints, and holy people of every religion have taught that when we forget our lives and serve others, then, and only then, do we find happiness. True joy is in the midst of life when we are present and of service.

There was a time in my earlier recovery when I looked at my life. I had been practicing twelve-step principles; I had been of service; I was showing up each day for meditation; I truly was trying to live a good life. Because of this, I really wanted a gold star next to my name, which would mean nothing "bad" would happen to me. What I didn't realize was that I had some wonderful challenges ahead of me that were going to change my life and give me even more peace and joy.

CHAPTER TEN

CHALLENGES/ GIFTS

In our earlier recovery, Tom M. and I used to say, "If it's this good now, what is it going to be like in another ten years?" Well, I must say it did and always does get better. We were anywhere from fourteen years to eighteen years in recovery when we started saying this, and we found ourselves saying that nothing bad has ever happened to us in our recovery. I could say this because of hindsight. Did I go through tremendous pain at times on the path? Yes I did, but in looking back, I could see where it led me. In hindsight, I could see the bigger picture. I could see that by staying in recovery and walking through whatever life presented, I grew from the experience. It would be like opening a door and walking from one room into a larger and more beautiful space—my inner abundance always expanded. The pain was simply an oddly wrapped gift.

My intentions are to quit labeling experiences good and bad, and to just melt into and embrace what is. When moving through life with an attitude of love about all things, I can move through each experience with tremendous peace and a smile on my face. To this day, with thirty-nine years in the program, I can honestly say nothing bad has ever happened in my recovery.

Without knowing it, in the early years I was starting to live a life based on the principle of equanimity. There is a story about equanimity; it is told in different ways, but here is a shortened version.

There was a village high in the Himalaya mountains. People living there were poor in worldly possessions. One day a herd of wild horses came running into the village and ended up in and old man's corral. Everyone gathered around and said, "Oh, you are so lucky."

He looked at them and said, "Maybe...maybe not."

Then his son tried to ride one of the horses, got thrown off, and broke his arm. Everyone said, "Oh, how unlucky."

The old man said, "Maybe...maybe not."

Then their village had to go to war with a neighboring village. All the young men in the village had to go fight, but the old man's son had a broken arm and didn't have to go. So everyone said, "Oh, so lucky!"

The old man said, "Maybe...maybe not."

This is the principle of equanimity in action: Move through our lives without labeling everything "good" or "bad." Life just is. There will be challenges. By grace, we stay on the path and then find ourselves looking at life with more compassion.

For example, when I went through the divorce around my thirteenth or fourteenth year, I doubted I could go on. I was in such pain. I can see now that if that hadn't happened, then I would never have met my current wife, Bea. My marriage to her has been the best thing that could have happened in my life.

Out of seemingly terrible events, such as divorce, come some of the greatest blessings. This truth has been reflected in the many challenges throughout my life. In 1999, my dad was dying of prostate cancer. He had been diagnosed with it about twelve years or so before and had had radiation treatments, but the cancer returned. I was in touch with my family through it all, and when my mom called and said, "I think you better come," I flew to San Diego right away. It was February 27, 1999. Hospice had been called in the week before. A hospital bed had been set up in the living room. Dad was drifting in and out of consciousness as I sat with him that day. I had gone through hospice training a number of years before, and I believe that the dying process can be beautiful in the spiritual sense, getting ready for the next adventure. I sat with him, and I told him it was okay to let go. As he lay there, slipping from this world to the next, I was talking to him. I told him that my mom, my sister, and I would be okay, and that he could move on now.

"Your body isn't working; it is time to let go," I murmured. Sitting on the side of the bed and holding his hand, where I had placed a Tibetan prayer bracelet blessed by Mother Teresa, I continued whispering in his ear, telling him to follow the light.

I asked, "Dad, do you see angels? Do you see the light?"

I had read so much of the dying experience and had heard stories from other hospice workers about the beautiful visions a dying person can see at the end. I was intent on helping my loving father cross over. All of a sudden, he became conscious. His eyes shot open and looked straight into mine with such fervor and intensity.

He declared, "Would you please shut up!"

In that moment I was shocked back to the realization of what a divine comedy life can really be. This is not what I expected, but it was perfect. Later that day, I was with my dad when he took his last breath and left. He did die with dignity, grace, and quiet.

About six months after my dad's passing, I went for my yearly checkup. One of the tests revealed my PSA levels were elevated— this is how they track prostate problems. Different blood tests were ordered, and a biopsy was taken to be sure. When my wife and I went to the doctor's office for the results of the biopsy, he sat us down and said the dreaded words, "You have cancer." His recommendation was to remove the prostate by surgery. We had caught it early enough, and there was a good chance it had not spread. I was stunned by the information I was receiving. I had cancer. He told me that with the removal of the prostate, there was close to 100 percent chance I would be incontinent. I would have no bladder control and would have to wear diapers. Also, I would most certainly become impotent. Yikes! Had I fantasized becoming a monk? Yes. Had I been celibate once? Yes. Were these still my desires, upon being married to this beautiful woman? NO. We thanked the doctor for his recommendation and walked out, never to return to his office again.

When we left, I was devastated. I had cancer, and my dad had just died of it. I told my son and cried a bit, but then after about two hours, I looked at my wife and said, "Wait just a minute here—nothing bad has ever happened in my recovery, so who says this is bad?"

Life has always had its ways of leading me to something better. Darkness and shadows also move through spectrums of pure light. I had just finished my Third Step with Bill the week before. In that process, I had made a decision to turn my life and will over to the care of God. That meant everything. The subject I was working the steps on this time was to learn more compassion. I became mindful of the fact that this was a wonderful way to feel compassion for others. All of a sudden, within two hours of finding out I had cancer, my wife and I said, "Okay, we are on the cancer adventure. Let's see where this leads us."

Bea looked at me and said, "Tom, one thing you have to know is I love you, and if you have to have surgery and as a result become impotent, you have to know in your heart I will never leave you. I will always be faithful; so let's move forward with this adventure." What a beautiful wife. What a support she was through it all, and to say those loving words to me in the beginning set the stage for what was to come.

We started doing research and discovered there was a new technique in prostate surgery called "nerve-sparing surgery." When they remove the prostate, if possible they leave the two bundles of nerves on each side. These nerves carry the blood flow to the penis, which gives a man an erection. The trouble was that this was fairly new surgery, and not every doctor did the procedure using this new technique. At this time, no doctor in Hawaii was willing to do it.

My friend Jack informed us that his brother had gone through this nerve-sparing surgery a year before. His brother happened to have the same insurance carrier I did and recommended a doctor in Los Angeles. The trouble with the healthcare system and HMOs is that you have to be referred to the specialist. Because I didn't have a referral from my primary care physician, his secretary wouldn't even put me through to him to let us talk. Somehow, though, I got his fax number and wrote a compelling letter about my situation. I included all the results of my biopsy, and let him know how important nerve-sparing surgery was to me. He called me immediately and gave us an appointment for consultation, so my wife and I flew to L.A. to meet with this remarkable doctor.

It was July when I found out I had prostate cancer, and in August I went into surgery. Bea and I flew to L.A. so I could have the operation. A couple of days prior to that, I was at a meeting and shared about what was going on with me. How blessed I felt to be on the cancer adventure. These types of things are challenges we have to face. In times like this, we can grow tremendously. Being mindful of each moment, we can walk through any event and come out the other side with so much light and love. At the end of the meeting, a lady approached me and said, "I feel like I'm supposed to congratulate you about having cancer. I have never heard anyone talk about it in this way."

During the period of being diagnosed and before going into surgery, I came to an understanding. It wasn't intellectual. This experience was heartfelt. A phrase presented itself in my consciousness: If you can't be happy now, then when? We have all these ideas of what will make us happy—more money, a relationship, a vacation, whatever it is. It is usually something in the future that might happen, and then when it does we will be happy. Yes, all those things can bring temporary happiness, but the key word is "temporary." The understanding that came to me was that happiness has to be right here, right now. Even with cancer, happiness and joy were mine to have with a peaceful mind if I was totally present for my life.

The day of the surgery, my wife and I arrived at the hospital in the early morning hours. My final minutes in the waiting room with her became like watching a movie. I had slipped into observing my present moment, without projection, anticipation, or fear. I found myself just being. As we sat together in the empty waiting room, we said nothing. Holding hands was enough. My name was called and they escorted me to the inner rooms of the hospital. The adventure was in progress. I had to have enemas to be cleaned out, and I was hooked up to a latticework of intravenous lines and clinical-looking cables. Normally patients are given a type of tranquilizer to calm the nerves. I politely declined. I wanted to be fully in the moment with no chemical distortion. I was breathing and being mindful of my breath to relax. When they rolled me into the operating room, I looked at everyone. Before they put the mask on that would knock me out, I said to everyone in the room, "You are all my angels today. I'm in your hands. Let's go for it."

When I came to after surgery, they informed me that they were able to save one bundle of nerves. They took no chances with the cancer and had to take out most of the other one, but thought they got it all. Within three weeks after surgery, I had complete bladder control. It took about eight months before the erection came back. When anyone inquires, I explain that it isn't what it was, but it's enough. I can't hang a towel on it, but hey, when I wake up in the morning, it is alive and well.

It has been more than ten years since surgery, and I'm still cancer-free. This is a total blessing. It has certainly led me to a place of more compassion for others having to go through any kind of illness and surgeries. I have reached out to others diagnosed with prostate cancer. I have also encouraged men to stay on top of their PSA tests. If detected early, prostate cancer has almost a 100 percent cure rate.

I also learned during this period, especially while waiting to see if an erection would still be possible, even more about impermanence in our lives, and about letting go. We are always letting go of things, especially the older we become. Bill pointed out that many of the teachers I had followed had lived lives of celibacy and had been totally fulfilled. So acceptance of what is had to become a real part of my spiritual life in those eight months.

I found indescribable comfort and great relief in the fact that Bea loved me, knowing that we would stay together no matter what. This only deepened our relationship. I'm not exactly sure what women go through with breast cancer, but I would think losing a breast would be something to be dealt with on a deep level involving womanhood. This seemed to be similar to what was happening with me. At times the feeling that I wasn't a man if I couldn't get an erection plagued me. This drove us to talk about sexual intimacy at a level we had not touched before. Sometimes the honesty stemming from these talks put my ego in place. It wasn't comfortable to find out how selfishly I might have approached sex in the past. Finding out I probably wasn't the best lover on the planet humbled me tremendously. For once I was really able to hear my wife's needs in this area. This elevated level of intimacy pulled us closer in ways that I could never have dreamed possible.

We will all have challenges. This is guaranteed. While here on the planet, in these bodies, living this life, challenges will come and go. There is a season for everything. Life has its ebb and flow. As we deepen our spiritual practice, we see the impermanence through these experiences. We learn to live with equanimity. Living by spiritual principles, we learn to walk through life with grace. We begin to look at the glass as half full instead of half empty. We begin to see a glimpse of what God sees, a constant yet gentle change based on endless possibility and benevolent wisdom.

The next few years proved the equanimity principle by knitting and weaving experiences into my psyche. Challenges continued to present themselves, and I was given many opportunities to practice staying present and trusting God.

In 2005, my painting company of fifty employees started to have financial problems. In the past, I was able to pull it out, but now we were much bigger. We were doing jobs of a million dollars-plus, and we were spread out on three different islands. I had given notice to my partners in the business that at the end of 2005, I wanted to retire from the company. With this intent, I asked one of them to get his contractor's license. One of these partners, who had been with me for many years, started drinking again. He was in charge of all the operations on Oahu. Our company just got too big and out of control. In the end, it collapsed under the weight of huge debt. By the end of 2005, the partner who had succumbed to alcohol left for California to go into treatment, which was great, but he also abandoned his portion of the debt.

On January 23, 2006, my wife and I were at a birthday party for one of her colleagues. Cool dance music from the sixties blasted through the room, though the dance floor was empty. I love to dance and sometimes get pretty wild. A great Earth, Wind & Fire song came on. I reached for Bea and said, "Let's go for it." She didn't want to, but I couldn't contain myself. I flew out on the dance floor and went wild. I was all over the place, jumping and having fun, when all of a sudden I came down and felt a distinctive pop near the bottom of my left leg. I could barely limp off the floor. I had severed my Achilles tendon. This event started a three-month ordeal in a cast.

This dancing injury occurred precisely two weeks before I was scheduled to leave for Thailand and India. I would be speaking in Thailand, but going to India first for a quick visit. My wife was scheduled to meet me in Thailand. We already had our tickets. So here I was on crutches, saying stubbornly, "I'm going anyway," even though the doctor had advised me not to go. I mean, it was an insane thought. Trying to maneuver the crowded streets of Kolkata on crutches was difficult at best and dangerous at worst, but I was determined.

However, on January 30 I was coming home from work, driving my SUV with a big cast on my left leg and my crutches perched in the back seat. Driving up Lama Street was my last memory. My next memory is someone waking me up in the car. A woman in an Indian sari was saying, "You have to get out of your car. It is smoking." Opening my eyes in complete confusion, I was surrounded by bits of a broken windshield, and the airbag was inflated on the passenger side. The car was totaled. I was repeating the words "What happened? What happened?" The ambulance and police arrived and helped remove me from the car. They placed me on a stretcher and put me in the ambulance. As we sped away with sirens blaring, I lay flat on my back, staring at the ceiling, thinking, "How did I end up here?" In that second, I saw how fast life could change.

Since I had been unconscious and had no memory of the accident, they took a CT scan of my head in the ER. Everything came back okay. After several hours, I was released. My wife had been notified and she took me home.

The universe had sent me a message, loud and clear. I had to cancel my trip to India and Thailand. As a result of the car accident, I was in great pain throughout my upper body, and navigating my way through the world on crutches became that much harder.

...gan going for acupuncture and to the chiropractor weekly ...e pain. I was having headaches that were getting worse, and I ...as thinking I was out of alignment, so I was getting chiropractic adjustments. In my morning meditations, I was practicing a Buddhist technique of breathing in my pain and also the pain of other sentient beings, then breathing out love and kindness for all. My head was really hurting, but I was getting some relief while in meditation.

Two months after the accident, I started doing weird things, like dialing the telephone and then walking away. I use the computer a lot, since I sponsor men around the world. Suddenly I couldn't even type a line without making all kinds of mistakes. Because my wife is trained in the area of human behavior, she became aware that something was very wrong with me. She spoke to my doctor, and he set up an MRI on Oahu. I had always had a car on that island because of the painting business, so I flew over and drove my car to the hospital for the MRI.

I hobbled through the hallways of the hospital on my crutches, finding my way to the check-in for the MRI procedure, thinking to myself once again, "How did I get here?" and wanting to ask, "Why me?" But I came back to my spiritual practice and tried to center myself in the present moment. I was laid on a moveable bed and told to lie absolutely still. I thought, "Okay. I can do this." The machine moved over me, and I just breathed, but I couldn't shake the feeling I might be on a movie set of *Star Trek*. When the procedure was over, they brought a wheelchair out and took me to the elevator to transport me to the floor above.

We got off the elevator, where the menacing sign that read "Neurosurgery" jumped off the wall at me. The doctor came out and calmly asked, "How did you get here?" I explained I flew from the Big Island, and then drove my car from the airport. He looked puzzled as he said, "We cannot even believe you can walk right now. You have so much bleeding in the brain that your brain has been pushed clear over to one side." He explained I had to be admitted immediately and scheduled for brain surgery first thing in the morning.

I called my wife right away and began to cry on the phone. I relayed the devastating information the doctor had just given me. I just couldn't believe it. She was very stable on the phone, and her steady demeanor calmed me.

I was hospitalized, and I called some friends on Oahu. My wife arrived on the island and reached the hospital by 7 p.m. When she walked in the room, there were ten people there. I had pictures of gurus and crystals all over the room. As she walked in, she declared, "This looks like a party!"

So we were on another adventure—the brain surgery one—along with the financial one. But we were in a good place, and we loved each other. That was the gift.

The next morning I was off to surgery. As I entered the operating room, the nurses all said, "April Fool's." So I will always remember the date was April 1. Doctors explained the procedure in detail. They intended to drill a hole through my skull, leaving a tube in to drain out the blood. I was given only a local anesthetic to numb the pain, so I was conscious throughout the whole ordeal. It was intense to hear and feel the vibration of the drill; it felt more like a jackhammer.

After the operation, I stayed in the hospital for a few days. Further CT scans revealed only 25 percent of the blood had been removed. Evidently, the problem had been going on too long, and the blood had started to coagulate.

The doctor said, "We are going to have to do a more invasive type of surgery." He explained that sometimes blood can break up and dissipate on its own, so I chose to go home for two weeks to see what would happen. I meditated every day and imagined the blood dissolving. I went back after two weeks to get a CT scan. The results showed the blood remained, so the doctor felt a more invasive surgery was necessary to remove the bits of coagulated blood. I was admitted at once for surgery. I called my wife again to tell her. One of my sponsees, Ted, was there with me, so he called other people for support. I went

...ry again, only this time they had to cut a four-inch portion ...my skull to clean out the blood. I needed general anesthesia for ...is operation.

I awakened in the intensive care room with my sponsor Bill standing nearby. As I came to, I remember mumbling to Bill, "What is this all about?"

He replied, "Tom, you are being tested and you are passing." Hearing this brought me to that place of acceptance of what is with another chance to just embrace and love what is. Suddenly, the room seemed to fill with peace. It penetrated my entire being as I lay powerless on the bed.

While recuperating from the brain surgery, I found a book in our house. It was by Pema Chodron, a western Buddhist nun. The title jumped out at me: *When Things Fall Apart*. There, I discovered an incredible message in the introduction of this book. Her teacher, the Venerable Chogyam Trungpa Rinpoche, said, "Chaos should be regarded as extremely good news."

Once again, the message is surrender. Always reach for surrender, which is the forerunner of the most beautiful peace and joy. We live in physical bodies on the planet Earth. We are in school, shall we say, and there is always homework to do. When mindful and present, we are able to complete our assignments and be ready for the next ones. There will always be a next one. And with each assignment, there will always be incredible lessons, like the message I got with my cancer: If you can't be happy now, then when? We begin to see the beauty and growth in all experiences that are put in our path when living in the present moment. In this most beautiful moment, we truly live in grace.

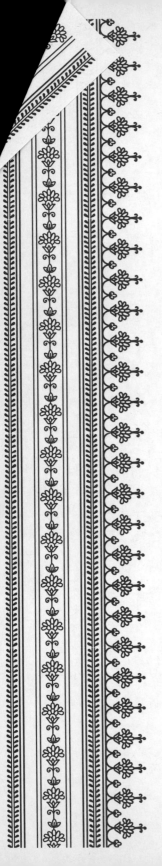

CHAPTER ELEVEN

HOLY PEOPLE AND SPIRITUAL EXPERIENCES

There are rock-and-roll groupies and movie star groupies, groupies for this and groupies for that. If I were a groupie, it would be for holy people and holy places. In my travels over the years I have made it a point to be in the presence of holy people or spiritually evolved souls. Whenever there was a chance of meeting one, I would make the effort to be there. Of course, I was blessed to be around Flobird for ten years. To be taught by someone who lived a life of giving love all the time, and to be actively involved in real-life miracles, is something I will never forget. Since those teachings and the passing of time, the parallel gift has been to be able to teach others the same gift of love and to participate in ongoing miracles.

His Holiness the Dalai Lama came to the Big Island of Hawaii in 1994 and gave a talk at Wood Valley Buddhist Temple. I volunteered

there off and on for about two months in preparation for
val. I repainted the temple with a crew of Tibetan monks as my
pers. What a wonderful time that was. On the day of his arrival, we
were honored to participate in a private ceremony where he blessed us
before the public was allowed access to him. These are just a few of the
gifts I would have never anticipated when I had first surrendered to
the path of recovery.

My wife and I also got to see him in his own home area of
Dharamsala, where we attended some lectures he gave. While there,
I got sick after a couple of days, and a western friend living there
arranged for me to see a Tibetan doctor. This doctor, we discovered,
was the Dalai Lama's personal physician. He gave me a physical in
Tibetan tradition, mostly reading the pulse, as they do in their practice.
He gave me some Tibetan medicine, which looked like little pellets.
I came back to our room, took the medication, and drifted to sleep
feeling quite sick. I had a vivid dream in which an old Tibetan woman
appeared to me. She seemed to be an ancient-looking holy woman. In
the dream I was standing up, and she was saying prayers while moving
her hands around my chest area. Then she dramatically pushed on my
chest, without really touching me, during the prayers. As she did this,
I fell over backward in slow motion to the ground. When I awakened
from the dream, I was totally healed, clear-headed, and feeling great. I
believe the woman was a Tibetan healer.

In 1999, several years after the Dalai Lama had visited the Wood
Valley Temple, a group of monks came to the Big Island. Traveling
with them was the Dalai Lama's personal medium. It is Tibetan
tradition for His Holiness to consult with an entity called the Oracle
on important decisions. In 1959 the Oracle was channeled and warned
the Dalai Lama to flee Tibet during the impending Chinese invasion
that claimed the country. The Oracle is channeled by an appointed
monk proclaimed to be the medium. The medium enters a trancelike
state to access the wisdom of the Oracle. Before going into this
altered state of consciousness, he is fitted with an elaborate headpiece

weighing somewhere around eighty pounds. Barely being able to stand while this is on his head, he slips into a trance as the ceremony begins, and amazingly, moves freely in a symbolic dance routine. As he moves around the floor, uttering messages being channeled from the Oracle, the messages are recorded for the Dalai Lama. This was the medium who was on the Big Island at Wood Valley, and we attended a public talk. After the talk, everyone lined up to be blessed. He had an artifact that was once stuck in a rock, which had been passed down to him from the previous medium. Shortly before the 1959 uprising in Tibet, the previous medium, his assistant, and other monks were led to some cliffs outside Lhasa. They discovered what they call a "revealed treasure." It was like a small dagger. It had been discovered when a pointed object was seen stuck in the rocks of the cliff. Knowing they had been led to this artifact, the monks tried to remove it, but no one could break it loose. Then the assistant to the medium put his hand down to try, and the artifact practically fell into his hands. This was seen as an indication that this holy treasure was intended for possession by the medium.

We all lined up, and as our turn came, we moved closer and sat before him. He moved this ancient artifact around our heads while saying prayers and gently touching us. When my turn came, I approached where the monk was seated in his colorful robes of deep burgundy and saffron. He was sitting against the background of a typically ornate and colorful Tibetan altar with golden Buddhas, gongs, and huge incense holders. I knelt down in front of him, and he started moving the instrument over my head. All of a sudden, vibrations of energy began moving through me, and I started crying. As he touched the instrument to my head, there was a loud cracking noise, like electricity popping. Everyone heard it. When I rose, I meandered into the back room and just sat there. I found myself feeling overwhelmed and in tears from the depth of the experience. The crying and vibrations continued for ten more minutes. When my wife came to check on me, she looked at my head and noticed a mysterious burn mark. I left immediately for home because I was in no shape to socialize that day. The monk even asked how I was. He knew something had happened in that moment. Given this experience, along with the Tibetan lady who came to me in a dream, my wife observed, "You sure have some strong reactions to the Tibetan Buddhist traditions."

I have several friends who are followers of Sai Baba, a holy man in India. It is said he can materialize things right out of the air. Mostly *"vibhuti,"* or sacred ash, is what manifests. With claims like this, there are many skeptics who say it is a trick. He has materialized many things for people—not just ash, but rings and other objects. You can have *darshan* with Sai Baba. This means being in the presence of a holy person and receiving the blessings. This opportunity happens each morning and afternoon at his ashram. On one of my many trips to India, I decided to witness this guru of so many people for myself. I was in South India at the time, and his ashram was about a three- or four-hour drive. Some Indian friends in the program drove me out. We all loaded into the car and drove through the countryside of rural India. After arriving in this small village, which was dominated by the presence of this holy man, we were led right to the ashram. Everyone was lining up for the afternoon *darshan*. We joined the line with hundreds of people outside a huge pavilion, waiting for the time to enter. As I followed the line of people inside, I found myself entering a beautiful structure supported by huge white columns. The entire floor area was made of marble. We filed in and took a seat on the floor. People filled the space to capacity while the silence overtook me. Stillness pervaded the room in anticipation of Baba's appearance. I looked up as he strolled into view with a long, saffron-colored robe and full afro hairdo. He almost looked as though he were floating along. From a distance, I watched as he moved through the crowd, stopping every so often to take notes that were handed to him, or waving his hand in the air to produce something that he would hand to a participant. At one point he was within ten feet of me when he waved his hand in the familiar way, produced something, and handed it to the devoted individual who held his hand out with great gratitude. Sai Baba has thousands of followers throughout the world. People travel to this small village in India because Baba never leaves India. He lives a simple life. He has helped India by building hospitals and schools, and by bringing clean water to rural areas throughout the country. My experience, from what I witnessed and felt within that day, is that Sai Baba is a true holy man.

My wife and I have been traveling to Bali since 1987. Indonesia is one of the largest Muslim countries in the world, yet the small Island of Bali is predominantly Hindu and Buddhist. This small Island of the Gods, as it is called, is an island of ceremonies. There are more holy days to be acknowledged than regular days in a calendar month. When moving about the country, even in the most crowded of streets, you must be mindful of where you walk. There are offerings placed in front of houses and businesses every morning. Little woven baskets with grains of rice, flower petals, and sticks of burning incense sprout up spontaneously, littering the walkways with humble offerings. You will also find them on the dashboard of every car. The Balinese celebrate their gods daily. Their spiritual actions aren't just compartmentalized into religious holidays and events. They seek the God of the moment. They move through their lives with smiles on their faces and love in their hearts.

Early one morning, before dawn, I was sitting on the veranda of our bungalow, listening to the sounds that one only hears while in a tropical setting—no cars going by, no sirens, just the sounds of the many species of life that surround you. I had an inspiration that I should start importing teak furniture and Buddha statues to Hawaii. I talked to my wife, and this idea was put into action. When we got home I talked to a friend, and he was up for being a partner in this endeavor.

We started doing business out of Bali in 1998, bringing beautiful items from Bali into Hawaii, which enabled us to fly in and out of the country three to four times a year. The twelve-step programs grew over the years with the expatriate community of surfers and other people in the export business. My good friend and business partner started living in Bali early on, after we started exporting teak furniture to Hawaii. He had been introduced to a Balinese holy man, considered to be an authentic healer. On one of our trips, he took me to this man's house. Houses in Bali are mostly open pavilions. There is usually a compound for family members, with these open structures surrounding a family temple. We drove to the outskirts of Kuta, which is about an hour's drive. As we entered the compound, I found myself in front of one of the pavilions. The older Balinese man was working on someone lying on a mat. He had a beautiful smile on his face, revealing a mostly toothless mouth. When it was my turn, I walked up the stairs and lay down on the mat, wearing only my shorts with no shirt. He began probing me, following some kind of map around my body, while giving attention to certain areas more than others. He giggled throughout the entire exam as his fingers seemed to dance over me, automatically knowing where to stop and bear down deeply, at times causing excruciating pain. I found myself jumping and crying out in pain, while all along he giggled or mumbled Indonesian incantations. Of course, I couldn't understand a word he was saying, but he certainly seemed to be having the time of his life at the expense of my body.

Our office assistant was there, so she translated some of what he was saying to me as he worked. I was astonished by his intuitive nature. He referenced things about my life he simply could not have known. This process of him giggling and me screaming and jumping around on the mat lasted for about thirty minutes. I thanked him and left a donation at an altar, where pictures of his Hindu guru peered out at me. This was one of the most bizarre "treatments" I had ever experienced.

The next morning I rose for my meditation before dawn. When the morning light became visible, I walked five minutes to the ocean. I had been a marathon runner for years, but had blown my knee out, so running had been replaced by early-morning walks on the wide expanse of beach. I especially enjoyed strolling along at low tide. Generally, I was able to slowly run for about five minutes at a time and then return to walking. On this beautiful morning, having received the strange healing treatment the day before, I started my morning walk. It was low tide, and miles of flat beach stretched out before me. Gazing at the waves and wading in the shallow, warm water of Bali, I began my short run. I jogged down the beach, smiling and saying good morning to other people who were also taking their morning walks. As I continued down the beach, watching dogs playing, and five male dogs hounding the one female in heat, I was lost in thought. Being mindful of my surroundings, I spotted a distant volcano rising up in the misty clouds. I was smelling incense from the offerings laid along the shoreline of the ocean when, like a jolt, the realization hit me that I had been running for quite a while. I noticed my knee had no pain, so after I turned around, I continued running the whole way back. I was acutely aware that while visiting the healer, I had experienced a spontaneous healing. My knee problem never appeared again.

Paramahansa Yogananda's book *Autobiography of a Yogi* had motivated me, even while still using drugs, to involve myself in the quest of the spiritual path and the practice of meditation. Throughout the early years of my recovery, I implemented some of the techniques of meditation I had learned while studying and being under the guidance of this great guru's teachings. In 1988, with about seventeen years in the program, I was led to return to his teachings and follow them to the end result of initiation into the practice of Kriya Yoga. Kriya focuses on mindfulness of the breath as a means for circulating energy up and down the spine. It takes about thirty seconds for one Kriya to be practiced. If performed correctly, it is believed to have the same effect as one year of common meditation. Being an addict and looking for the instant rush, I was immediately intrigued. My wife and I both started receiving the meditation lessons I had first received in 1966. Although we had both been meditating for years, we started on lesson one. This process went on for three years. The lessons are intended to advance you deeply in meditative practice until you are ready for the Kriya ceremony. Once we had completed the requirements to receive the Kriya initiation, we flew to Los Angeles, California, to attend the ceremony of practicing Kriya meditation. We filed into an auditorium with about one hundred other devotees. The SRF monks gave talks on this ancient practice. We received personal assistance from the monks on the proper breathing technique of Kriya meditation. We both left this ritual, or rite of passage, with the feeling that this was one of the most important things we had done together, ranking it along with the day we were married.

The other book that made an incredible impact on me was *Be Here Now* by Ram Dass (formally known as Richard Alpert) and Tim Leary. Reading this book after I got clean, I saw it as a story by two addicts, Tim and Richard. Tim continued using, but Richard went to India, which for him was akin to entering a twelve-step program. He met his guru there and discovered that on the truly spiritual path, we don't need drugs. He came back as Ram Dass, and his story of transformation was much like many of ours in the program. We found out that truly living a spiritual life doesn't involve getting high. Ram Dass had a stroke in the mid-1990s that left him in a wheelchair. By being mindful in his life and staying in the now, he found acceptance in his life. He lives by the principle of equanimity. He has said that he has never been more grateful and at peace than in the last few years; this is coming from someone who can't get out of a wheelchair, but has found great joy in his life. After I had the brain surgery, my wife and I got an invitation to visit Ram Dass on Maui, where he lives now. We spent the afternoon at his house, and he truly is a loving and gentle soul. My personalized license plate on my car reads BHRNOW.

I read a book a few years ago called *Cave in the Snow* by Vicki Mackenzie about Tenzin Palmo, a western lady who became a Buddhist nun. She spent twelve years in retreat in the Himalaya mountains. This book touched me deeply. I must have bought ten copies to give to others. To be in solitude that long was so inspirational to me. I have done many silent retreats, but to consider silence for twelve years is astounding. My wife and I traveled to Northern India to Dharamsala, the home of the Dalai Lama, where all the Buddhists who left Tibet have sanctuary. While there, I had the book with me, and was talking to the nuns about Tenzin Palmo. Within a few days, one of the nuns came running to our room and said, "Tenzin is here. She is getting ready to leave, but she will be at the bus stop in an hour." Like magnets, we were pulled from our room and propelled down the hill. Carrying her book with us, we found her. Her mission since leaving her place of retreat high in the mountains has been to establish a center for women to develop a spiritual practice leading toward enlightenment. She was in Northern India in search of land. She was very receptive to our excitement. I found my elation hard to contain, gushing about how much I loved the book and that I had bought so many copies to give away. She found this funny, and joked that I should travel with her to promote her cause. Bea and I had our picture taken with her, and she also signed our book.

Retreats are certainly something to consider for anyone with a sincere practice of meditation. I'm certainly not suggesting twelve years in a cave in the Himalaya for everyone. Retreats come in an assortment of sizes and formats, from one day to three months. When I say "retreat," it is in the context of an organized get-together with a retreat leader or meditation teacher. Many people make the excuse that there isn't enough time. Even a daily practice, doing morning meditation, has many citing the lack-of-time excuse. The truth is that the busier we are, the more important it is to meditate on a daily basis. There are many one-day retreats where forty-five minutes to an hour of sitting is followed by teachings, and then participants sit again in silence. This type of retreat also usually involves mindful walking as a form of meditation. My wife and I both have attended many retreats, from one day to ten days. I have found them all beneficial. I believe that creating a space empty of mindless chatter while having extended periods of meditation punctuated by spiritual teachings is such a boost to spiritual development. Most retreats require silence, no eye contact with others, no books, and no writing materials. Even the one-day retreats are practiced in silence, except when teaching is in session and questions may be asked.

The goal is to just practice going into the silence. Books, pens, and paper are distractions from the process. I have found that longer retreats give space to finally slow down and become comfortable. Removing oneself from daily activities sets the stage for spiritual connection.

After three days, a settling in seems to take over. Our "busy self" finds a way to give up. Over the years in my practice of meditation, I have learned that showing up and expecting nothing is the key. The simplicity of following my breath, noting my thoughts and body sensations, isn't always easy. Expecting guidance, desiring to see the third eye, wanting a bright light, or yearning for any type of transcendental experience just causes suffering. The lesson is to sit, listen, and experience what comes up.

As I have shared, guidance has come in my practice, and I base my life on this guidance, but it doesn't happen every day. I just practice. I have read about people's experiences, like what happened to Flobird on the beach when the universe turned to light and love rushed through her, or with Bill W., the founder of Alcoholics Anonymous, in his hospital room. He had a similar experience of a blinding light and a transcendence that brought on the profound experience of him not drinking again. I call those movie-type awakenings. This type of spiritual experience is not necessary and won't happen to most of us. In twelve-step programs, as with other paths, the awakenings come slowly. Yet as we look back, we see the change in our lives. At the time of this writing, I have been doing some form of meditation for forty years. Thirty-seven of those have been while in recovery. I have mentioned those times I have had experiences of guidance. I have had my third eye revealed on many occasions. Many times I have gone so deep, I'm sure my breathing has come to a place of almost stopping, and the peace and stillness has been profound. Hearing the sound of silence in these places is riveting, but most of the time the practice consists of watching the breath and watching the thoughts. This is practicing mindfulness, and it is the beginning of enlightenment for us all. To be caught in the moment is beyond explanation.

A few years ago, I was on a ten-day silent retreat. The daily schedule started at 4 a.m. and ended at 9 p.m. The first meditation took place between 4:30 a.m. and 6:30 a.m. Then breakfast was served, and meditation resumed again by 8 a.m. The total meditation time during the day totaled twelve hours of practice. On the seventh morning of this routine, I arose and sat for my first two-hour meditation. After breakfast I sat in a chair outside my tent, waiting for the ringing of the bell signaling the next practice. Then we would all take our places in the meditation hall, which was actually just a large, circuslike tent.

There were around thirty men and women participating in this retreat. As I sat in silence in the chair next to my tent, I found myself staring at the blades of grass beneath my chair. I noticed the vast amount of movement taking place. Small bugs were scurrying around, busy with their lives. I looked up at the tree I sat beneath. It was as though it had summoned my attention; it was calling out to me, and I could feel its living energy. I became so mindful of the life forces surrounding me, and the thought came to me that I'm never alone. Even if I was on a deserted island somewhere in the middle of the ocean, I would never be alone. There is just so much life around us at all times. As I sat there, tears began to roll down my cheeks, and I felt so much love and oneness in that moment. The gong sounded, and I took my place in the meditation hall.

Previously, on the fourth day of this retreat, I had started experiencing a soft, peaceful flow that swept through my body. From the top of my head, it would float down through my torso and out my feet. This peaceful flow of energy came every time I became still enough to notice it. As we began our second session on the seventh morning, I continued to feel this peace finding its way through my body. It was so pleasant, but I would just notice it, without attempting to grab on and try to keep it. Just being mindful of it was enough. Within about twenty minutes, a tear found its way down my face. The feeling of oneness I had experienced while waiting for meditation to start welled up in me again. I found myself acutely aware of the thirty other sentient beings sitting with me in this practice. It was as though I could feel everyone's inner strivings. Waves of compassion and love began running through me with such intensity that tears readily streamed down my face. My nose was running, and I could barely contain myself. The silence was broken by the sound of sobs that came pouring out of me. Vibrations emanated through me with such magnitude I actually felt paralyzed in position. I knew if someone were to touch me they might feel the electricity that seemed to be coursing though my body. I felt as if there were thousands of volts flowing through my every cell. This energy seemed to continue for twenty minutes, as did my sobbing with love and compassion for everyone, knowing we were all connected, feeling everyone's joy and their suffering. Without warning, this thundering vibration multiplied ten times in strength as it rushed up my spine, exploding at every *chakra*. *Chakras* are spiritual energy centers located at various points on the body, with several positioned along the spine.

The vibration moved to the base of my head, with a final eruption blowing out between my eyebrows as the energy found its release. I sat there in amazement at what had just taken place, knowing in that moment that I had done nothing to ignite this experience. I had no power; it has always been grace. The teacher asked me to come forward. It took another five minutes before I was able to get up and walk to him. I sat in front of him. Instead of saying to the remaining students, "See what can happen when you keep up your practice? You too can have these wonderful experiences," he whispered to me, calming me down. Without excitement, he made it clear that I should not get attached to this experience. These things happen, but they are just experiences, and to crave them and look for them is to cause suffering. This reminds me of things I have heard like "When you find out you're God, go chop wood and carry the water," or "After the ecstasy, do the laundry."

To live a life that is full of joy, a life that we can move through with a deep peace, we must reach for equanimity in all things. This also applies to spiritual experiences or awakenings along the way. Suffering is caused by our cravings and aversions, as the Buddha taught. To crave always for things on the outer, or even crave for things on the inner, like profound experiences in meditation, only causes us to suffer. That is the nature of desire. Also, our aversion to pain causes suffering. When we are running from something, we can find no peace. Looking back over my life, I reach for hindsight, noting things I might label as bad. When I embrace it, practicing being in the moment has led me to real joy. Like the farmer in the Himalaya when the horses came running into his property, we look at life with the so-called good and the so-called bad, and say, "Maybe...maybe not."

CHAPTER TWELVE

THE PRACTICE, THE DHARMA

Once we have stepped upon this spiritual path, it becomes our *dharma,* meaning our "life's work." As our practice deepens, we discover that our reason for being here on Earth is to ultimately serve others with complete abandon.

When I first begin a relationship of sponsoring someone in the program, whether they have been clean for a few months or have been in the program for twenty-plus years, my first question is: "What are you doing with your Eleventh Step?" In a way I am simply asking them, "How is your relationship with the present moment?" This step is the most critical facet of the program. It is surprising how many people do not have an everyday practice. I suggest starting with ten minutes each morning by finding a place to sit each day. I further suggest creating an altar with pictures or items that touch the individual spirit. Begin by simply showing up each day for ten minutes. This will become a habit, and this habit will become the practice. We must remember we are all practicing each day. Even His Holiness the Dalai Lama shows up for his practice. We are always becoming.

Our goal in life is to serve, but also to be present as we do this. We try to become aware of compassion and eventually find ourselves practicing compassionate awareness. We can learn to be present by sitting down and following our breath as it goes in and goes out. As we feel the air in our nostrils, often our minds will wander. The mind will have thoughts. That is what it is designed to do. Like the ocean with its waves, the mind's process is natural. Allowing the thoughts to come and go, we return to the breath. If we keep up the discipline and simply be patient and gentle with our attempts, we will eventually exhaust our ego, and when it is trying to "catch its breath," we find stillness and the essence of our true nature moving in time with our inhalations. When in the breath, we are in the moment. This is our practice. We learn to observe ourselves as we move through our lives. Every day, with every movement, we try to be present. When we walk, we truly walk. When we are driving, we are right there, driving. We learn to be present by paying full attention to the daily routines that we normally never think of. Being mindful of everything we do is the practice. We can then find joy in each instance, like the time I bent over to take a drink from a hose on a hot, sunny day. I found myself just drinking the water while feeling the warm sun on my bare back. This experience became so full of love and joy that I burst into tears. We can have this even while washing the dishes. The practice of being mindful in the moment can be like making love, if one is truly washing the dishes.

What I have found to be true is that life is exciting. I will never be retired. I will never be bored or with nothing to do because I have this beautiful practice. As long as I have a breath to follow, I have a way to stay present. There is really nowhere to go, because we are already here. The destination is this moment, and we have already arrived. There is nothing complicated about this. The simplicity of finding ecstasy right here, right now is magical.

My *dharma* is to live my life to the fullest each moment. Flobird taught us to always give love and to find a way to put love into action every moment. Getting out of the self and thinking of others is the key to unlocking all of the love in the universe. It is here in infinite abundance. To awaken each morning with the thought of "What can I do for someone else today?" is the goal. How can we ever think we have nothing to do, with all the people running around our planet who need love? We have such a gift to give in each moment.

Without waking up in the morning to the habit of meditation, there is no way I can find the strength to live such a life of action. We all must find time each day to go within. This is where the power to live life to the fullest comes from. The ten minutes of meditation will expand as our practice develops. In this quiet time each morning, we find the guidance and the strength to live a life of service. These principles once again are something we always walk toward. We find direction when we simply ask. Humility is patient action. We will never be perfect. That is why it is called a practice. The gift is our birthright. We are simply strolling toward it, enjoying the present view.

As our *dharma* unfolds, we all will be shaped by our own unique experiences. These experiences are where we will find the willingness to continue on the path and keep growing and changing. The Twelve Steps are always there, marking the path as we move forward. Every time we reach out to love someone without a price tag, our passion of loving every sentient being will grow.

We will never be alone on this path. I used to think, "if I'm not around Flobird, how can I live?" But I have since realized that we are always sent dharma teachers, sponsors, gurus, or whatever you want to call them. They will come our way if we keep our hearts open. The teachings are everywhere, especially in times of great challenges. If we remain open with our thoughts, remain in the present and in service, and embrace a love for life, then we are always right where we belong.

If anyone happens to call Bea's and my home and gets our answering machine, he or she is greeted with a message stating that we are out living and loving our lives to the fullest. That is exactly what my wife and I try to do. Living life to the fullest means we are embracing each moment of the day. Sometimes we are at the beach; sometimes we are making love; and sometimes we may even be having brain surgery. Loving every event with passion and presence is possible.

Remember, there are only two things that ultimately motivate humans in this life: fear and love. Why not choose to be motivated in each moment by love? Believe me, the fear will try to creep in, and when you let it in, fear will bring all its friends. Anger, resentment, jealousy, depression, and an endless list of negative emotions can accompany it. These are the children of fear, and are feelings that separate us from one another. If we continue our practice of meditation and service by coming back to the moment, we find that in the moment the whole universe is on our side. We discover that love is what holds it all together. God is loving us now.

CHAPTER THIRTEEN

THE STEPS*

I was first introduced to the Twelve Steps after going to my first meeting held at Flobird's house on the North Shore of Oahu in 1968. Today, there are hundreds of twelve-step programs based on the original twelve-step concept launched by Alcoholics Anonymous in 1935. The steps are basically the same for each of these programs, except for the First Step, which begins with "We are powerless over…" You can fill in the blank with "drugs," "alcohol," "food," "gambling," etc. I use the word "addiction" when referring to this step, because it encompasses all unhealthy obsessions.

In the early 1930s, a hopeless alcoholic sought help from Carl Jung, a well-known psychiatrist. The patient had resigned himself to the tormented reality that he suffered from the chronic inability to

---

*Reprinted by permission of NA World Services, Inc. All rights reserved; Twelve Steps reprinted for adaptation by permission of AA World Services, Inc.

stop drinking. In those days, such people often ended up in jail or a mental institution, and many lost everything that had ever been dear to them, including family, friends, careers, and, ultimately, life itself. Addiction was viewed as a lapse in morality and had not yet been recognized as a medical disease.

This man came to Dr. Jung and asked for help. The psychiatrist frankly told him that although he was unable to help him, he had—on a few rare occasions—seen someone in the grips of alcoholism go through a profound personality change brought on by an intense spiritual experience. The steps were designed to achieve the kind of spiritual experience that brings on the deep personality changes in our lives to which Dr. Jung referred. One could argue that the steps were "given" to addicts by a higher spiritual realm, and Jung was an observer of the truth that the recovery movement would come to believe. In his later years, Jung would be asked if he believed in God. Jung reportedly answered, "I *know* there is a God." Yet the experience of working and living the steps can be as varied as those seeking recovery, and belief in a theistic god or God Itself is not a requirement. Spiritual principles work for the agnostic as well as atheist. The process simply asks us to believe in something, some Higher Power that we will be willing to let guide us on this journey of healing.

Sponsorship is highly suggested in all twelve-step programs. When asking someone to be your sponsor, you look for someone who reflects in life what you are seeking. This person will guide you through the step process—someone you can call in a time of confusion, someone you trust spiritually.

Each of the steps contains certain spiritual principles. Some twelve-step literature emphasizes the HOW of the program. This acronym refers to three basic principles: Honesty, Open-mindedness, and Willingness. There is a deliberate order and harmony in the way that each principle is placed, practiced, and ultimately lived within the twelve-step process. As we work these steps, our lives begin to change. We are transformed by these principles "from the inside out," and as our spirits heal and grow our material lives are positively changed. The serenity that is spoken of so highly in twelve-step fellowships flows outward, attracting others who seek it out. We write out each step, identifying what the step means to us and how it applies to our lives today. This process is similar to a Zen master giving his student a Koan to figure out and solve in his or her life. The most famous example of these playful, mystical riddles would surely be: "What is the sound of one hand clapping?" The student then meditates on this phrase (or step) to come up with what this means personally and spiritually in his or her present life.

Since our spiritual journey involves constant change, we continue to grow by working the steps over and over again, each time on a different issue and at a deeper level. The journey of the steps mirrors our lives, and their meanings change with us over time. The principles that occur as we work and live the steps are, quite simply, directions. Like points on a compass, they tell us where to go, directing our lives into a place of wholeness and fulfillment. I believe this profound personality change has to be ongoing. To assure that our transformation continues, I suggest to the people I sponsor that they keep their practice of the steps ongoing. The steps save our lives, and then they change our lives. We, in turn, show the next person how we did it. Ideally, this process of spiritual growth never ends.

STEP ONE

We admitted that we were powerless over our addiction,
that our lives had become unmanageable.

An honest working of the First Step requires a personal admission of powerlessness over alcohol, drugs, or other addictive behaviors. The Buddha gave us the four noble truths; the first is in alignment with our First Step, the reality and admission of our inherent suffering.

Like any path, the spiritual path begins with the First Step. We addicts of the hopeless variety are fortunate to have Twelve Steps that, when worked in the order they were written, offer guidance about what to do next. We must embrace each step and work it to the best of our ability in order to be ready to move on to the next one. If they are not practiced in this orderly fashion, the steps lose their power to create miracles that bring freedom and change our lives.

In addition to helping us get honest, Step One is designed to bring about surrender. I don't believe we can go forward on any spiritual path without making a decision to quit fighting everything and everybody—even ourselves. We must come to a place where we are willing to give up, to allow our selfish ego to get out of the way. We allow the magic in.

Step One requires the admission of hopelessness and defeat, an acknowledgment that our willpower is insufficient to overcome our addiction. Why have we consistently failed to change the mess of our current lives using our own power? The First Step provides important clues to this dilemma and prepares us for the work ahead.

If we surrender with real honesty and go to a deep place inside, we are left with a feeling of hopelessness that is depressing and painful. But this situation is actually beneficial, although it may not seem that way when we are in the middle of it. We are no longer resigning ourselves to the comfort of denial. Our true powerlessness is now a palpable and actualized thing, made real by our deepening practice of surrender. As long as we continue to hang onto any hope that we are capable of changing ourselves, that we can regain the willpower to beat our addiction, we are doomed to fail.

As long as we maintain the delusion that we can cleverly manipulate our lives to get what we want, the miracle is diminished or impossible. If not promptly addressed, this illusion of self-sufficiency may well lead us right back out of the program. Once again, we must reach for surrender, admit our powerlessness, and get our egos out of the way. Step One is where grace can enter our lives.

The First Step leads us to an acceptance of our addiction problem. Who wants to admit this? That's why it is imperative that we be beaten down (or reach a bottom) to allow this grace to enter our lives.

As a newcomer to the program, I found myself in an uncomfortable state of vulnerability brought on largely by the results of my addiction, including the loss of money, family, friends, and self-esteem. I had destroyed everything around me, and Step One made it possible for me to make this admission. The rawness of my now-drug-free body, combined with the clarity and awareness that guided my mind and spirit, brought the unmanageability of my life into a blinding focus.

Even those with long-term recovery whose lives have become remarkably successful must be willing to work Step One over any new problems that arise. We must continue to reach deep within and find a new surrender to our current situation. The spiritual path constantly calls for us to get out of the way.

It is a spiritual axiom that everything in life is impermanent, which means there is nothing to hang onto or make us feel whole at all times; alcohol, drugs, overeating, sex, gambling—whatever the addiction—eventually stops working. The fortunate ones are given the gift of hitting bottom. That emptiness is a product of our true powerlessness. To discover this is a gift because it leads to greater peace and acceptance.

Sadly, if the problem is unaddressed, many find their bottom is the grave.

Despite wealth, fame, and accomplishments, all human beings are subject to impermanence. People, places, and material things will always come and go; we can't stop it. There are times when we will be stripped of everything we have tried to hold onto. Once we accept those seemingly unacceptable circumstances, we will be led to surrender; and on the other side of surrender is a joy and peace that is not of this world. This is what we are offered if we follow the spiritual path. After surrendering through the First Step, our once-shaken spirits are at times calmed by a quiet sense of hope, and we become ready for the next step.

STEP TWO

We came to believe that a power greater than ourselves could restore us to sanity.

Step One begins the sometimes dark journey within, pushing us toward the truth of our powerlessness and hopelessness, leading us to the principle of surrender. Left with just Step One, we would continue to live in a state of desperation. This First Step is quite simply stating the problem. In many ways, it is our only problem: a pure sense of powerlessness combined with a now-blatant awareness of our unmanageability. This despair can be our friend, for now we can turn the page of a new life and find Step Two. This step introduces us to the idea of a power greater than ourselves, the message being that we can be restored to sanity. In writing out the steps, we always talk about where we currently are on our spiritual path. Depending upon our length of recovery, we have different issues to work on. Thus we must always stay current with the particular step we are working. Step Two says "restore us to sanity." Does that mean we have been insane? My guess is yes; at some level we have been insane.

I define sanity as living in a place of love, living in the present moment. Insanity occurs when we are living in fear and separation. This consciousness comes from living completely out of the moment when dealing with situations in life, meaning there is no reality to the way I'm processing what I'm going through. The second noble truth the Buddha taught is that we see the cause of our suffering, which is our desire or craving for attachment. This simply translates to addiction, and accepting this moves us toward sanity.

When I'm separated from the moment, I'm out there doing it all by myself. Our Higher Power only lives in the present moment and can only guide us in the here and now. When we project about something in the future, we are actually making it all up. We have no idea what any outcome will be, so our mind is running a thousand scenarios that are all fantasies. Once again, we are trying to control the world around us, projecting an imagined power over reality. And yet again we become emotionally unmanageable, and eventually may act out or use yet again. This is truly insanity. When not present in the moment, we find ourselves in fear. Fear and love, it has been said, are the only two states of mind that motivate us. Which is the saner choice to make?

One of the spiritual principles that come up for me in Step Two is trust. I have to look at my insanity and the powerlessness I admitted in Step One. I have to ask myself—and it may not be easy— why would I resist coming to believe when I'm feeling so separated from everything?

This is when we look at the deep surrender that we found in Step One and realize that we need to find a way to trust. Often that means we must look around at others in recovery and see the program working in their lives. Even if we cannot experience the presence in our own lives, we can see it working all around us. We can come to believe by looking at the sanity in their lives. We begin to learn and trust the twelve-step process of recovery.

The deeper our surrender, the easier it is to achieve trust and allow it to become part of our daily experience. We may not yet see a way out of our addiction, but we know that, left to our own power and warped thinking, we have failed miserably. We have nowhere to turn but to a power outside our own ego. This power is the force that illuminates our once-darkened and forgotten spiritual path.

In Step Two, we use the words "Higher Power" rather than "God." Many people new to a twelve-step program have some old ideas about God. It is a word that can turn some people off, and they might choose not to continue with recovery via the Twelve Steps.

This is the step where the newcomer, or someone with multiple years clean, can change their concept of God. Whatever concept of God was not working up to this point can be altered. This is important even for the person who has long-term recovery. We tell the new person to "come to believe" that there is a power outside themselves, and that they must form a relationship with this power. It does not have to be the fear-based, patriarchal God, or the punishing concept of God that they were raised with. In a world of presupposed and alleged freedoms, this may be the ultimate freedom—the freedom to believe. The Twelve Steps are about that initial and recurring surrender. To keep a pointless war going on inside about that controversial and misunderstood word, God, will only hinder true grace from entering. An open mind will elevate our being and a Higher Power will hold us aloft.

We work with our sponsor on these issues, and we listen to what others in recovery have to say about them in meetings. Some are advised to sit and watch the ocean, which is a power greater than us. Many find comfort in this. Some of us have been told we are going to hell if we do anything pleasurable. We have to let go of these old dogmatic and punitive ideas of this judgmental type of power. It's a slow process, but by feeling love from others in our twelve-step meetings, we begin to awaken.

Each time we practice the steps and the principles they embody, we grow along spiritual lines. As we incorporate the steps into our lives, profound personality changes continue to occur. Deep within, we begin to feel something positive working by doing Step Two. We put trust into action and begin to feel hope. We are now beginning the journey of awakening.

STEP THREE

We made a decision to turn our will and our lives over to the care of God as we understood Him.

The first three steps are the foundation we are building to let go of our ego and maintain our spiritual journey. In Step One, we began our surrender. In Step Two, we moved in the direction of coming to believe that a power greater than ourselves could enter our lives and begin the process of change.

Step Three asks us to make the decision to turn everything over to God. Some of us who have had a negative reaction to the word "God" are now able to begin to move on and let a new relationship unfold. The twelve-step literature tells us that this God can be of our own understanding. Some people call it "Good Orderly Direction" (or, more humorously, "Group of Druggies" or "Group of Drunks"), and some might simply call it Mother Nature. The Buddha called it right view. The third noble truth the Buddha taught was the end of suffering: nonattachment, letting go, turning it all over.

As we walk through each step with our sponsor, we begin to see how the steps were divinely written and arranged in perfect order. By the time we have entered the Third Step we are gradually sensing or "intuiting" a beneficial presence and sense of relief in our lives. Each step, when completed, prepares us for the next one. It may feel as if doors are opened and new possibilities are revealed. The first three steps help remove or retire our ego, or self-will. Making the decision to hand our life over to the care of our Higher Power is like sidestepping our self-will and letting us become open, for only then can grace begin to enter our heart and soul.

Step Eleven is where we find the guidance and power to carry out the decision we make in Step Three, but this cannot happen until the preceding ten steps have paved the way to a newfound freedom. The Third Step is where we allow a loving and ultimately liberating Higher

Power to guide us through life and direct us through the subsequent steps. It is like discovering the equivalent of spiritual electricity. It is one of the most transcendent decisions we will ever make.

Some of the principles involved in Step Three include surrender, trust, and faith. Here we are asked to surrender at an even deeper level, but we are shown that there is guidance in this surrender. So it is faith that helps us to abandon ourselves to the care of a loving Higher Power with whom we are developing a relationship. In some ways, the Third Step is about making confident choices and decisions, however mundane or important they may be, and having faith that we are making the right move. We trust that we are no longer alone in the universe, and God is working directly in our lives.

When I started going to meetings in the late 1960s, I remember listening to an older man who talked about the process of Step Three, the turning over of our will and our lives to the care of this power. "Give us ninety days, and at the end of ninety days, if you want it all back, you can have it," he pointed out. "You can have the depression; the waking up in your own vomit, so sick you cannot move; the lying in the gutter; losing your family, friends, and money. Yes, you can have it all back."

So when we look at what we are really turning over, especially during the beginning of our journey, is this really so hard to do? We are turning over a life that wasn't working; otherwise, we would never have been led to the program. It usually takes a huge upheaval to get us to this realization. In some ways, our struggle with Step Three is laughable. We have nothing to lose and everything to gain.

Step Three is an interwoven and conscious part or our daily practice of Step Eleven. It involves being mindful of giving our life to our Higher Power every day, sometimes several times a day. This allows us to be totally aware of and open to guidance from our Higher Power. When things are going badly, we can be still and calm for a moment, breathe in and breathe out, and give all of our pain, indecision, and suffering back to God. Pausing to do Step Three during our busy day allows us to let go of our burdens.

For some of us, this will be the first time that we have experienced the feeling of not being alone with our own inner war. This is a revelatory moment in our once-solitary and isolated lives. We learn that we don't have to walk through life by ourselves, that we have a miraculous process that leads us away from chaos toward freedom.

The fourth noble truth from the Buddha is the eight-fold path— by following it we can be free of suffering. The eight-fold path is encompassed in the remaining steps: right understanding, right thought, right speech, right action, right livelihood, right effort, right mindfulness, and right concentration. You will find all these principles in the steps and more.

The way to complete Step Three is to move on to Step Four.

STEP FOUR

We made a searching and fearless moral inventory of ourselves.

This step can't be stated more clearly: searching and fearless. You can't rationalize this simple direction. It means dig in and get it all out. We aren't talking war stories; we're talking feelings. One of the principles underlying this step is courage, as is self-honesty.

Most twelve-step books offer some type of format on how to work Step Four, including outlines and lists of questions to be answered. The truth is that there is no wrong way to do this, as long we just start to write.

I was told from the beginning of my recovery to write my emotional life story, and to really focus on examining the feelings behind all my life dramas. This step is the first clue in the investigation of our very essence, and the detective work begins with putting words on a page.

One reason many recovering addicts end up in therapy is because we have stuffed awkward feelings and alien emotions for our entire lives. The first time I was rejected by someone, my reflex was to bury those feelings. I did not remember them and was not even conscious of them. In Step Four, I gradually started to uncover all of those seemingly lost yet still-uncomfortable emotions. These feelings of rejection and hurt were buried in my heart; so every time I was rejected, those same feelings would bubble up to the surface, over and over again. If we have not admitted and released these feelings through the steps, we are at high risk for relapse. It is a sad prophecy that many in recovery who never work Step Four and take this inventory will relapse and use, again and again. If nothing else, simply that dire fact should help generate the courage and honest introspection needed to carry us through this stage of the steps.

Working Step Four begins the process whereby we take an active role in our recovery. We really start to work. This is why we say "work" the steps. It won't always be easy or comfortable—we are ready to uncover, discover, and recover.

Writing out Step Four, we put everything on paper. Gradually, we begin to see the patterns that were established when we were very young. Some of us lived in dysfunctional family situations, so healthy role models were absent. On the other hand, some of us grew up in fairly healthy families, but still we got messages that there was something wrong with us. Despite our childhood circumstances, we now need to take responsibility for our recovery. We have been led to the Twelve Steps, and this process can take us to freedom. It is not uncommon for many newcomers to mistakenly think that we are "alone" in writing the inventory. They forget that we can talk to our sponsor or another in recovery who has worked this step. We surrendered our will and lives in Step Three; our Higher Power is right here with us as we write, providing the courage and self-honesty we need. Many deepen the practice of prayer in this step, asking for strength and guidance before beginning their actual writing.

I was asked in the beginning of working the steps to write down all my fears, and to write my story on paper. If I had trouble getting started, it was suggested that I write about the incidents I would never reveal to anyone, the ones that would find me choosing death rather than reveal them. Believe me, after doing this the words readily began to flow. Once you write down the worst thing you think you ever did, it becomes easier to let the pen fly across the paper.

Step Four is called a moral inventory. Initially, it focuses on the hurtful, embarrassing things that we have done or have had done to us. This can be an extremely painful experience, but this buried garbage has to come out. A positive way to look at it is that the steps are introducing us to new principles that allow us to lead a better life, but first we have to be cleaned out, tossing out our old ideas about people, places, and things. We must be emptied out so there is room within for the new life to grow and blossom. Most importantly, many forget that Step Four is quite simply things that have already happened. It is not some nefarious "to do list." These things are the past. We are simply putting them all down on paper.

As the years of recovery begin to build, we find ourselves going through the steps even when we are feeling good. Then Step Four can focus on assets, not just our liabilities. Some say the first time they did a moral inventory it was difficult to write about their positive attributes and actions. But a Step Four moral inventory calls for the good as well as the bad.

Sometimes we can write our Step Four in one sitting, which could take hours to complete. But I have also seen longer inventories done over the course of several days. The key is to get it out and then go on to Step Five. The longer we prolong this process of writing our inventory, the longer we are sitting in the pain of emotions that are arising. This is especially true with newcomers. Feeling all these raw emotions over an extended period of time is not easy. But our sponsor once again lovingly reminds us that while we work this step, we are reliving our past. Therefore, the sooner we finish our writing, the sooner we can "give it away" in Step Five.

When we are writing Step Four, it's a good idea to avoid reading it over again every time we sit down. We simply just keep writing. The intent is not to rationalize or analyze what we have written. There is no wrong or right way to do any of the steps; the point is to just trust this proven process and quite simply to work them.

STEP FIVE

We admitted to God, to ourselves, and to another human being the exact nature of our wrongs.

When I first started going to meetings, I heard it said many times that you can do Step Five with anyone, which is true. Some people might feel more comfortable with a priest or therapist; but in my own personal experience, I believe that it's best to take this step with your sponsor, who has already gone through the previous steps with you.

In Steps Four and Five, we get in touch with the exact nature of our wrongs. Usually, the person listening to our Fifth Step writes down our character defects and lists various people and situations that would be part of our subsequent Eighth Step. This is why it might be important to walk through all the steps with your sponsor. He or she has already walked this path and can help in making it less confusing and awkward for you. When looking for a sponsor, be wise about the person you choose. When I first started coming around to meetings, there were people who told me to "look for the person you are most scared of and then ask him to be your sponsor." I now see that they were trying to explain that what "bothers" me about someone may mean I actually share the same personal qualities and traits. I felt then and still feel today that ideally, a desired sponsor should simply be someone who "has" what you want. This could be something as basic and worldly as a successful record as a businessperson, or an admirable ability to maintain loving relationships with others, or even a more transcendent quality of serenity, selflessness, and pragmatic wisdom. As sponsor and sponsee work the steps together, a closer and more intimate relationship develops. The writing of Step Four and then the admission made in Step Five are in some ways the crux and cornerstone of this highly intimate bond based on the highest levels of personal respect, integrity, and trust. This is the reason it is recommended that men work with men and women work with women, because of this almost inevitably deep intimacy that will develop.

People in meetings often talk about the freedom they experience after doing the Fourth and Fifth Steps. While this is true, sometimes we are also left with a painful dilemma. There truly is an indescribable freedom in the sense that we have finally revealed all of our painful secrets; but we are also likely to experience many uncomfortable emotions and feelings related to our defects of character. How do we deal with it? We move on to Step Six.

Steps Six through Nine will deal with the personal pain generated by admitting our character defects and realizing the harm we have done to people, places, and things over the course of our lives. We then make our apologies, make our amends, and start living our lives in a more proactive and positive manner. They are the healing steps. With our sponsor's guidance, as we move through these steps, freedom will certainly rise from the depths of our now-healing spirits. With the admission of this step, many of us are surprised at how much we now truly want to grow. We find ourselves getting ready to change our lives with the willingness found in Step Six.

STEP SIX

We were entirely ready to have God
remove all these defects of character.

After finishing the Fifth Step with our sponsor, we will receive feedback and, hopefully, a list of our character defects and harmful behavior patterns. This helps us to see the exact nature of our wrongs.

A character defect, in most cases, is a normal character trait gone awry. Take fear, for example. It's appropriate to be fearful while walking down a street at night and seeing a gang of thugs ahead of you. That fear would prompt you to take a certainly healthy caution and head in another direction. On the other hand, living with daily irrational fear is an overreaction that cuts you off from leading a healthy, peaceful life.

Another example is lust. You can have lust in many areas of your life, but most of the time if it is listed as a defect, it is attached to sex. It is a natural energy running through our bodies that we can use in a healthy and positive way, such as to maintain a long-term relationship that includes an exciting and active sex life. However, if you are sneaking around your neighbors' yard peeking into their windows, we can safely say that your sexual drive has surely crossed the line from a natural instinct to a defect of character.

When first reading this step, most people think, "Of course I'm ready to have these defects removed. Why wouldn't I be?" But when we look at it in an honest way, it's not that simple. A defect of character can also be considered a survival skill that we have used for our entire lives up to this point to get whatever we have wanted. We must ask ourselves: "What am I getting out of this defect? Is it working in my life?" The truth is that people are not really willing to let go of certain behaviors if they are still working beneficially in their lives. So we must search deep inside ourselves to honestly answer these questions. Sometimes the answers may be painful, but we simply need to ask our Higher Power for the willingness to change and let go of these behaviors and defects, however ingrained they may be in our lives.

Step Six requires that we go deep within to honestly acknowledge our defects and investigate the patterns we discovered in Step Five. Then we must ask ourselves, "Am I ready to let go of this defect, or am I still getting something out of it?" We will want to take a thorough look at this list and go back in our lives to identify when the defect first arose, how it benefited us in the past, how long it has persisted, and how it can eventually harm us and other people. Now, with our newfound spiritual path, we can decide if the defect nurtures us and the people around us. If not, then maybe we are willing to finally let it go.

STEP SEVEN
We humbly asked Him to remove our shortcomings.

There's an ongoing controversy about the difference between a "shortcoming" and a "character defect." To me, they refer to the same thing. I once heard an audiotape by Bill W., the founder of AA, who was the acknowledged channel for writing the Twelve Steps, wherein he said he simply didn't want to use the same word again. Some people use the analogy that a character defect is having a flat tire and the shortcoming occurs when we drive on the tire. Regardless of the wording, we are ultimately speaking of the same negative traits.

Steps Four through Seven are about seeking a deep personality change and truly changing who we are. This change is a spiritual transformation. This central process within the Twelve Steps could be outlined quite simply as this: In Step Four, we write out what we did. In Step Five, we admit that we did it. In Step Six, we realize that we no longer want to do these things. In Step Seven, we ask God to help us. Or, even more simply, "This is what I did; this is why I did it; I don't want to do it; so God, please help me."

The key word in this step is "humbly." Step Seven says, "We humbly ask…" Before approaching this step, I suggest defining humility to yourself in silence with your Higher Power. Through the years, the meaning of humility might change for you. I ask my sponsees to write down the definition and then go ask three people they respect spiritually to define the term. After reviewing their comments, analyze your original definition of humility and make any changes as needed.

So, just how do we "humbly ask" our Higher Power to have our shortcomings removed? This step, like the Third and the Sixth Step, usually takes place during morning prayers and meditation. Flobird used to say, "I always ask to remove these shortcomings in my meditation; I leave the results up to God." This is a daily program, and we approach life day by day. So we are humbly asking God to help us today in removing these fear-based and destructive beliefs and behaviors.

In this process, we realize that we never had any power of our own to change. If we had this power, why would we even need the spiritual path of the Twelve Steps? This is why we approach Step Seven with humility. Humility is simply knowing I have no power; it is God, a Higher Power, love, or the universe working through me. I always remind my sponsees that if they have any doubt that God will remove these shortcomings, they need only remember that He has already removed the ultimate defect. "What is that?" they will invariably ask. I then remind them, "The using itself."

The initial humility we practice when we first come into recovery is only intensified through the working of the previous steps. In Step Seven we realize that we do want change, and we practice humility by now knowing that only God can change us. So we are merely channels, a reflection of a loving God's grace, and by doing these steps we are clearing away the blocks between us and our Higher Power. Then we can become more open and clear about just why we are on the planet—to follow our inner guidance and to be of service. This humility and realization lead us in now wanting to correct any harm we may have caused in our addiction, so we now can move further on our journey toward Step Eight.

STEP EIGHT

We made a list of all persons we had harmed,
and became willing to make amends to them all.

As with our list of defects, we also have a list of amends that arises from doing the Fifth Step with our sponsor. When we get this list, we take it home and begin to add names or situations that later come to mind. Our sponsor will then help us clarify and then decide whom we put on our actual list.

At this point, many people find it quite difficult to separate the Eighth and Ninth Steps. Step Eight is simply a list of the people, places, or institutions we have harmed in any way. We make this list without thought of the amends that will follow. We must stay focused on what Step Eight is asking us to do, which is only to compile the list and to pray for the willingness to make the amends. We will find ourselves projecting about certain amends. We just keep coming back to the list. We try not to imagine how the actual amends will play out and what will happen. If we are consumed with worry, we can speak to our sponsor or another in recovery and also remind ourselves that God has us in Step Eight—not Step Nine. When we mentally "time travel," it is so painful because we go there alone. God is here in the present moment, giving us the willingness and forgiveness to work Step Eight. This willingness is very important for our spiritual growth, and, of course it offers us some assurance of not going back to whatever addictive behavior brought us to a twelve-step program. We can also find comfort in knowing that the list in Step Eight is similar to the writing of Step Four. Once again, we don't pontificate or "theorize" about this step; we simply do it. We make the list! We work this step, and we write it out.

Our sponsor should be a part of this process; he or she can help by arranging the list in a simple order, the easy ones first and the harder ones toward the end. Our willingness at this point is what we have come to know so well in our approach to staying clean. Willingness is one of our key spiritual principles.

STEP NINE

We made direct amends to such people wherever possible, except when to do so would injure them or others.

When working closely with our sponsor and discussing our amends, we might discover that perhaps making some amends could cause harm to others. We must always remember that when making amends, our ultimate goal is to heal old wounds and not create any new injuries. Step Nine advises us not to make particular direct amends in certain cases. This concern is usually for the other person and not us.

This is where guidance from someone we trust who has experience with this step is crucially important. It's dangerous to be so excited about the promise of being free from addiction and guilt that we run out and begin madly making amends. We don't start this delicate amends process by saying "I'm sorry" to everyone in sight or start blindly giving out money to everyone we owe or think we may somehow owe. It's important to follow the list, and perhaps even more importantly, the experience and directions from our sponsor.

When I got clean on the North Shore in 1971, Flobird and her birds were far away on their adventure in Egypt, and Tom M. was on Maui. I was excited about being clean and was preparing to leave Hawaii for California to take my son to his mother. I was selling things to raise money for an airline ticket. I found myself feeling guilty and troubled because I owed $65 to a woman I had been buying heroin from.

Like a typical addict making amends with no direction from a sponsor, I went to her house and paid her the $65. In retrospect, she would not be on my amends list. And going to a drug dealer's house when I only had a few days clean and money in my pocket was not a smart thing to do. I'm lucky I didn't use again. I am lucky to have survived that "amend." This is a strong and possibly life-threatening example of why we follow directions and don't go off to do amends on our own, even though our motives may be confused as healthy.

In addition to willingness, another important spiritual principle is forgiveness. So much spirituality in this life is based around this principle. There are two ways that forgiveness works in Step Nine. Making amends to people does not mean we are just telling them we are sorry for our behavior. We may have forgotten that many of us made countless apologies in active addiction, yet would simply repeat the same destructive moves. Our apologies may be in question to those closest to us and those we repeatedly have harmed. To make amends means to change. True change always requires some type of corrective action. We now live our lives differently, and much of this difference involves correcting the harm we have caused, and, just as importantly, no longer harming ourselves and others.

When we make direct amends, it is wonderful if the person offers immediate forgiveness. If this happens, our relationship with that person begins to heal almost immediately. But there will be times when he or she might not want to see us or even hear about the situation again. Perhaps we have totally alienated people with our past behavior, and they now want nothing more to do with us. We must be willing to accept whatever occurs, and remember that God is working with us in Step Nine, not against us. God will move mountains, but we need to bring our shovel.

Even if our amends are not accepted, something profound happens within us. The willingness we have been given in the face of adversity gives us the grace to forgive ourselves, and this is what really counts when the forgiveness comes from within. When we can forgive ourselves, we begin to live with a peaceful heart. This now-illuminated heart encourages us to no longer hurt ourselves or anyone else. This is what Step Nine is about. Forgiveness is an action based on the highest realms of love. It is so much more then simply saying, "I'm sorry." It is amending the behavior and starting to move through life with a more gentle and loving spirit. This is the wondrous gift of the Ninth Step.

This willingness is the gift that allows true healing to begin. We must be willing to make every amends on our list, even if it means we may go to jail. There will be times when our sponsor says not to make a certain amends for whatever reason or circumstance; we follow that direction, as we have followed direction and continually walked forward with the willingness, courage, and trust to do anything we must to stay clean. This is where the magic comes from, by living a life based on spiritual principles.

Some people experience their first real freedom in the program after the Fifth Step, but most experience it after the Ninth Step. The healing that occurs and the God-consciousness we begin to feel may take on an almost supernatural hue. By the end of this step, we have cleaned up, or attempted to clean up, a lot of the wreckage of our past. This is a turning point for most people in a twelve-step recovery program. They have courageously acknowledged their actions and the harm done to others, and have been willing to do something about it. We now learn to monitor our newly invigorated spirits in Step Ten.

STEP TEN

We continued to take personal inventory,
and when we were wrong promptly admitted it.

When I first saw this step I realized the message was that we have to continuously work on ourselves, and that self-examination is ongoing in the spiritual life. I remember in my first year of recovery I read a statement from the twelve-step literature that helped me realize that any spiritual disturbance I am experiencing, the problem is within me. For me, this meant I had to stop blaming others for my thoughts and actions. What a wake-up call this was. Myriad thoughts and reasons poured through my mind, trying to convince me this couldn't be true. As the acceptance of this realization began to filter through my rebellious soul and then gradually settled within me, I embraced this new truth. I then knew that if I truly wanted peace in my life, I would have to live the principle of mindfulness to a greater degree. I had to pay attention to the eruptions of feelings that followed me constantly everywhere I went. When I felt disturbed, I would have to go within and find out why. All feelings are open doors. In Step Ten we learn to walk inside them and see exactly where we are in the present moment.

I kept a journal for more than twenty years of my recovery. With daily writing I became in touch with my feelings, and my open-mindedness and actual openness grew with the continued practice of this step. Denial was no longer an option when I detected anything that threw me off-balance. I had to address it, and the sooner I did, the better I felt. This step acts as an ongoing barometer which sounds an alarm that directs us to look within when we are disturbed and to practice self-examination and mindfulness. We now know that no one can "make us" feel or do anything. We have an inner consciousness and conscience and a Higher Power that now aids us in self-awareness.

Last year I was in line at the bank, where I had gone for years and assumed everyone knew me. My turn at the teller window came up. The young woman behind the teller window was new. She did not know I was once an owner of two businesses and was held with high respect at this particular establishment. I handed her my check. She then shyly informed me that it was over her assigned and allowed limit, and she would have to get approval. This delay in my very important day would have not occurred with a teller who knew me and knew of my "importance." I would have been in and out of the bank in my usual record time. When the teller returned after what seemed like an interminable wait, I was a bit impatient and not as understanding as I should have been. I was simmering in my anger. My emotions had once again betrayed me, clouding reality. After all, the poor woman was simply in training. I had yet again "personalized" an essentially mundane and normal daily inconvenience.

This diseased reaction did not assume the form of anger or rudeness, but quite honestly, I just wasn't being compassionate and kind. As I left the bank and was walking to my car, I felt disturbed, and that inner barometer went off. Call it a Higher Power or a healthy conscience, but I knew that I was bothered by what had just occurred inside that bank. I got in my car and sat there, staring at my hands resting on the steering wheel. Gently closing my eyes, I came back to my breathing; I came back to the present moment. I took a personal inventory in that moment, looking at my feelings and motivations. I knew then that I had to go back to the bank and make my amends to the teller. That meant I had to wait in line again, but I made the amends. It really made her day, and it made my day once again joyful and peaceful. To an outsider "looking in," this may seem like a pointless or even frivolous gesture. But the process of the Twelve Steps is guided by a higher, ethereal realm that may seem illogical or weird at first glance. The ultimate dividend on this simple investment of my time was that she appreciated my forgiveness, and I in turn felt clear. The step process absolutely works.

Some people call Steps Ten, Eleven, and Twelve the maintenance steps. I just call them the steps, and in my view, I have to continue working all twelve. My spiritual path contains twelve steps.

Knowing that Step Eleven involves meditation, it's obvious I cannot sit in meditation if I am disturbed. So the pure function of Step Ten is to keep us from running movies in our heads as we sit for our Eleventh Step. Step Ten could be seen as preparing our soul and spirit for prayer and meditation by being mindful of any distractions that may impede our desired closeness with a Higher Power. Again and again, our attention is drawn to the divine order that the steps are in.

STEP ELEVEN

We sought through prayer and meditation to improve
our conscious contact with God as we understood Him, praying only
for knowledge of His will for us and the power to carry that out.

Over the many years of putting the steps into action in my own life, I have arrived at the conclusion that Step Eleven is the center of the program. It is the endless source of spiritual strength and the vortex of an otherworldly energy. All the work we have done in the prior steps has prepared us to go within and connect with a Higher Power. Remember when Carl Jung told his alcoholic patient that in a few rare instances he had seen people like him go through a profound personality change brought on by a spiritual experience? That was the flashpoint of a Higher Power, the big bang of recovery. The Eleventh Step, the practice of prayer and meditation, is the vehicle within. Through the practice of this step, we let our breath transport us to the quiet place within. If calmly called upon, this inner place can freely guide us through the rest of our lives.

The Eleventh Step is where Step Three finds its completion. In the first three steps, we discovered that we had no power and had to get out of the way. We turned our lives and our will over to this power. Now, in Step Eleven, we are seeking knowledge of this power's will for us—and the strength and ability to carry it out.

There are two important things to keep in mind about the way Step Eleven is worded. The step says we are seeking to "improve our conscious contact," meaning that we are not going to perfect this task. The word "improve" implies that we have already had some form of contact with a Higher Power, and by the time we get to the Eleventh Step, the events and miraculous changes in our lives should be evident. This is a form of conscious contact. It is also a practice we follow daily. We must practice the principle of discipline daily to achieve this contact. Anything positive that we practice regularly will lead to self-improvement, and so it is with Step Eleven.

The other part of the step says that we "pray only for knowledge of His will for us." Nowhere does it say we pray for a relationship, a new car, or more money—just the simplicity of "His will for us." This is difficult to do in times of a crisis. My tendency is to always ask, beg, or plead for whatever it is I think I need. Flobird always told us to follow any prayer with "Thy Will Be Done." This neutralizes my longing for things that may or may not be good for me. Living this spiritual life means embracing a life of surrender, and in that surrender I am acknowledging that I have no idea what needs to unfold spiritually in my life. So in the Eleventh Step we are seeking knowledge, and then, on some level, an understanding of what God wants us to do. We don't need to know *why* we are to do something. We need only know *what* we are supposed to do. God has the power. We are simply seeking knowledge of that power and the strength to act on it.

I have learned to sit in meditation. I let the breath go in and out, and I just let my thoughts be thoughts, letting my desires for certain things to manifest in my life come and go. I don't have to beg or plead. I just let the intention be there and follow it with "Thy Will Be Done." I have found that the universe is for me, not against me. Love is all there is. All good things and abundance will come my way if I just let it happen.

The twelve-step programs don't teach meditation; they just give a simple suggestion in the Eleventh Step that perhaps our sponsors or others can help us with this. There are many books on meditation, and some will resonate with you while others will not. Go with what feels comfortable; we are following this twelve-step practice for a lifetime. There's no easier or softer way. We just have to keep showing up for the practice.

People pick sponsors in the program whom they respect and are drawn to, learning to trust their guidance and suggestions. I prefer to have a sponsee start out with at least ten minutes a day of meditation. Since there are twenty-four hours in a day, you can sit for ten minutes and let God know you care. Of course, we can increase this time, but it is important to start the practice, start the discipline, and simply show up. Soon meditation will become a habit, and you won't want to skip a day.

It is also important to set up a place to meditate. Going to the same place each time creates a vibration in that area of your house, outside, or wherever you feel most comfortable. When you approach this spot you begin to feel relaxed. You can light candles and incense if you wish, look at pictures of holy people, or create some kind of altar that consists of things that make you feel good. So many things can contribute to your practice. It becomes a lifestyle.

Until we can become intimate with this power, we cannot be fully intimate with others. The disease of addiction is a disease of separation. Recovery from addiction is about creating intimacy in our lives, going within and being intimate with God, our higher self, love—whatever you want to call it. This is the path to intimacy with others.

STEP TWELVE

Having had a spiritual awakening as the result of these steps,
we tried to carry this message to addicts and to
practice these principles in all our affairs.

Remember being in school, reading a book, and then having to write a report on it? Step Twelve is that book report. After working the first eleven steps, it says that as a result of working the steps, we have had a spiritual awakening. Don't complicate this statement. It says what it means. The spirit within us awakens. We carry this message to other addicts, alcoholics, overeaters, gamblers, whatever the addiction may be. The message is the spiritual awakening. Through this spiritual awakening, people seeking recovery can experience a profound personality change. This step also says that "we practice these principles in *all* our affairs."

The Twelfth Step is not only the summary of what the steps are about, but it also points us in the direction that can lead to complete fulfillment. The Twelfth Step calls us into service. For some newcomers, the Twelfth Step will be one of the first times in many years that we have thought of helping others. We begin to realize that our life depends on our ability to get out of self and serve others. This is a profound realization, transformation, and awakening in itself.

The step tells us we need to carry this message to other addicts. We have to give away what has been so freely given to us, or we won't be able to live a life free from addiction. Step Twelve also says we must practice the principles of the steps in all of our affairs, meaning inside and outside the programs. The intention is to become fully aware that we are spiritual beings having a human experience.

It may be hard for us when we are first called upon to give of ourselves. Maybe we have to go out of our way to give a newcomer a ride to a meeting, or go to coffee with someone after a meeting because they want to talk or they are hurting in some way. But these simple acts of selflessness will start to become common. Paradoxically, our sense of peace and comfort in being in our own skin deepens as we deepen our spiritual practice and seek guidance from a Higher Power. We find more joy here as we try to contact "there." And whatever a Higher Power or God may be, it seems to compel us to help others. The constant refrain in countless faiths, religions, and mystical quests is nearly always the same: prayer and meditation combined with the practice of selfless service to others. The twelve-step path, being a spiritual path, is no different.

Our lives begin to change dramatically as a result of working the steps, beyond our own limited view and imagination. As we begin to study the many spiritual books that will find their way to us, we discover once again that service to others is a huge part of the peace we find through living a spiritual life.

People in the program are extremely lucky. We have a disease that, if kept active, can destroy our families, our jobs, and even our lives; so we can't sit on the fence. There is no such thing as a partial surrender. As we work these principles in our lives, the spiritual life becomes something achievable, not just something we read about in books or hear a guru talk about. It becomes something that we long for and are willing to go to any lengths to live. Surely, we are blessed. We now share the blessing.